SOME ASSEMBLY REQUIRED

A True Story of Love and Organ Transplants

TJ CONDON

Black Rose Writing | Texas

First printing

Some names and identifying details have been changed to protect the privacy of individuals.

ISBN: 978-1-68433-736-1
PUBLISHED BY BLACK ROSE WRITING
www.blackrosewriting.com

Printed in the United States of America
Suggested Retail Price (SRP) $18.95

Some Assembly Required is printed in Book Antiqua

*As a planet-friendly publisher, Black Rose Writing does its best to eliminate unnecessary waste to reduce paper usage and energy costs, while never compromising the reading experience. As a result, the final word count vs. page count may not meet common expectations.

For Jim, you resilient badass.

Praise for
SOME ASSEMBLY REQUIRED

"*Some Assembly Required* is an honest, funny, heartwarming look at resilience in the face of illness."
–Christina Consolino, author of *Rewrite the Stars*

"As the family member of a transplant patient, I can say, *Some Assembly Required*, is a beautiful and educational resource for transplant patients and their support group."
–Timothy Sojka, author of the *Payback Jack*

"TJ Condon has written a very powerful and intimate account of the tremendous challenges faced by the loved ones of those struggling with illnesses that require organ transplantation.
I couldn't stop reading it!"
–Dr. Alessandro Bartoletti, author

SOME
ASSEMBLY
REQUIRED

PREFACE

This book is not intended as a substitute for the medical advice of physicians. The reader should regularly consult a physician in matters relating to their health and particularly regarding any symptoms that may require diagnosis or medical attention, for goodness' sake!

I have tried to recreate events and conversations from notes and memories. Most names and some identifying details to protect the privacy of individuals, because even exceptional people sometimes have thoughtless moments or bad days. But, since this book celebrates and chronicles one couple's truly crappy *year*, neither this author nor her husband can luxuriate in anonymity.

CHAPTER 1: EARLY JUNE

Our House, Central NJ

"I think I need to go the emergency room," Jim said, a pained expression on his face.

"Didn't you just see the doctor?" I asked.

"Yeah, but this isn't right."

Jim had just returned from a trip to the grocery store with no groceries.

"I parked the car, got out and started walking inside. But I thought if I walked all the way to frozen foods, I might not make it back."

I looked hard at him. My husband was not usually the melodramatic type, so I figured this might be his flu talking. Mostly I couldn't help but deduce that I wouldn't be getting the ice cream I had wanted.

"Maybe just try resting for a bit?"

"I don't think that will help." Jim lifted his shirt. The skin of his belly looked as if it was stretched tightly across an overturned salad bowl. It was as if someone had dared Jim to swallow a basketball and/or toddler.

"Does it hurt?"

"It feels...I don't know, exactly. Taut. Yeah, taut is the word."

I started weighing my options. Was his condition unusual? A bit. Was it "Emergency Room worthy?" Maybe. I had my doubts, but at a minimum I supposed "in sickness and in health" meant accompanying one's spouse to the ER upon request.

"Okay," I sighed. "Let me grab my stuff and we'll head over."

Jim had felt lousy for the last few months and really truly bad for the past few weeks.

It was as if he, and therefore we, were living under a gigantic black cloud. First, Jim's employment contract ran out, and they declined to renew. Then his mom died a few months later. While Jim was working to settle her estate, his doctor diagnosed him with type-2 diabetes. Next up was this new and unknown malady.

About two weeks before the ill-fated grocery trip, Jim had gone to see our primary care physician. Following some blood tests, the doctors sent Jim for an ultrasound. After checking out the results, the doctor referred Jim to a specialist. The problem was, this specialist was so special Jim couldn't get an appointment for weeks. He still had no official diagnosis.

"Can you help me with my shoes?" Jim asked, snapping me back to attention.

"What did you just wear to the store?"

"Loafers. I want to wear my sneakers."

I rooted around the bottom of his closet and found a pair. I unlaced them and handed them over to him, thinking the job complete.

"No," Jim said awkwardly. "I mean, can you help me put them on?"

"You can't do it?"

"No. I can't bend over to tie them."

"Because you are in pain or because you can't reach?"

"Both. But mostly the second one."

I tugged them over his swollen feet and laced them up.

"Did you just do double bunny ears?" He asked teasingly.

"Yeah. It's the only way I know how to tie shoes." I retorted, daring him to keep poking.

He held out his arms, and I pulled him off the bed and into a standing position. It took a bit of doing; Jim was not a slim man. He had been steadily gaining weight over the past year. He wasn't in *"needs a crane to get out of the house"* territory, but honestly, he was on the way. He lumbered more than walked, and he constantly complained of a sore back and creaky knees. The shoe help added insult to injury. I didn't want to be the lady who had to put shoes on her corpulent husband.

As he shuffled his way to the garage, I handed him the keys.

Jim drove.

That was our family's most steadfast division of labor. I worked and did laundry. Jim drove and paid the bills. Even in his condition, he wouldn't think of offering me the keys and I wouldn't think of asking.

He wedged himself into the driver's seat. I helped him slide the seat back even further than usual so he could fit. His arms barely reached the wheel over his belly.

For the first time since the early days of our dating, I knew I had to ask:

"Are you really okay to drive?"

"Yeah. Yeah," Jim shooed me away to the passenger seat.

We made the 15-minute drive to the hospital in silence. Then, we parked in the closest available space and made our way to the parking garage elevator. Jim was unsteady on his feet. I held his hand and pushed the elevator button.

Hospital, Emergency Room Waiting Area

We had a choice of two emergency rooms. One was where Jim's father had stayed during his long illness. The other was where his mother had stayed for hers. We chose the mom hospital because we knew the layout and thought the nurses were nice.

We lived near a city—close enough to enjoy the benefits of great doctors and excellent restaurants, but far enough to live a suburban existence. The hospital was in the middle of the city, so an everyday ER visit might include, say, a gunshot wound. By this point, however, it was early afternoon on a Sunday. Any Saturday night excitement had passed, and those left in the Emergency Room didn't have dramatic symptoms—a feverish kid here, a juicy-sounding cough over there.

Then there was us.

From a triage perspective, Jim was clinically uninteresting. No shortness of breath. No heart issues. None of the *FACE* stroke symptoms. No puking. No crapping his brains out. Not even a low-grade fever. He was just tired and couldn't touch his toes.

As he answered the nurse's questions, I filled out the insurance forms. I figured the $500 Emergency Room copay would earn us a few minutes of a highly qualified physician's time to examine Jim's big, round belly and tell us he was super-constipated. If what Jim needed to ease his worried mind was paying the equivalent of three fancy dinners out to be told to take a massive crap, so be it.

Not that I lacked sympathy; I was just plain exhausted.

I'd recently taken on additional responsibilities at work, and they included a lot of travel. I worked for a defense and aerospace company, which meant I spent 90% of my time traveling to and from purposefully unmemorable locations that I never got to see much of, anyway. This was the first Sunday in three straight months I wasn't on a plane and/or packing a bag. It was to be a day of rest, dedicated to the fine art of extreme loafing. It seemed both Jim and the universe had other plans.

The nurse showed Jim to a bed, handed him a gown and tugged the curtain closed. I once again leaned in to help him with his shoes.

We waited.

A Bookstore Coffee Shop, 11 Years Ago

Jim and I met on Match.com.

Our first date was in late December, during that space between Christmas and New Year's reserved for being lazy and eating leftover cookies.

For me, dating had largely been a volume game. I liked to plan things in five-year increments. If I got married at age 25, I could then have kids by age 30.

I had just passed the 24-and-a half mark and was well on my way to unrecoverable spinsterhood. Earlier in the month, I'd made a commitment to myself. If I was going the Old Maid route, I'd best do it the modern way—by getting a master's degree. My New Year's resolution would be to give up dating for the foreseeable future.

When I got an email alert on Christmas Eve from a guy on Match.com who suggested we meet, it surprised me.

Dammit. I thought. *Hadn't I turned that off?*

I looked for an excuse to say no, but then curiosity got the best of me. I read his profile and saw an interesting tidbit about a Swedish pancake pan.

Apparently when he visited out-of-town family for the holidays, he made them breakfast in said pan.

My mind wandered to images of a strapping Swede standing at my small apartment stove, flipping tiny hotcakes on a lazy Sunday. *Could there also be bacon?* I read on.

His post felt breezy when it was difficult to pull off breezy. Back in those days, you had to entice would-be mates with a maximum of words and minimum of pictures. He had brown hair and bright blue eyes. The single picture he'd offered featured him standing confidently at the top of a mountain, his hands on his hips as he looked straight at the camera with a beautiful sunset behind him. He looked like the poster child for self-actualization.

The pancake pan and confident-looking picture attracted me. The absence of spelling and grammatical errors sealed the deal. He had set my English major heart ablaze.

Why not make this guy my dating grand finale? I thought. After this, which had to be my 53rd blind date, I would officially hang up my spurs.

I wrote back and gave him a choice of meeting places, either a nearby bar or a bookstore/coffee shop combo. He went with option two.

Suddenly, there we were.

I had just sat down and was contemplating what to order when in walked a man with hair more reddish than in his photo and a set of perfect teeth. We'd both arrived a few minutes before the appointed time and, what can I say, his punctuality was sexy.

He wore a sweater and leather jacket combination that made him look super cute. I would later learn his preferred attire was 10-year-old T-shirts bought on sale. I would also learn that his friends— intimately familiar with Jim's t-shirt collection—dispatched one of their kindly wives to take him wardrobe shopping so his dates wouldn't think he was approaching them in Starbucks to beg for cash.

We introduced ourselves, and he asked if I wanted a coffee. Before I could make my request for a decaf, non-fat with two pumps of no-sugar vanilla, he went up the counter and returned with two extra-large drip coffees with ample room for milk. I was strictly a *"no caffeine after 10 a.m."* gal, and it was now past 8 o'clock in the evening. Not wanting to be rude, I thanked him for the coffee and braced myself for a sleepless night.

"So, tell me about yourself," he said as we settled into our seats.

"There's a lot to tell," I warned.

"How about the basics?"

"Well, I work in marketing. [In a job I loathed—I left that part out.] I grew up in New Jersey and have lived here all my life, except when I went to college in Pennsylvania. So, what do you do?"

"I'm an attorney."

"What kind of law do you practice?"

"Municipal law," he smiled. "Contracts and stuff."

I liked that he wasn't braggy.

"Where do you live?" I continued my questioning.

"Across the street."

"Seriously?"

"It only took me and my car 15 minutes and three jug handles. I can point to my apartment."

Okay. So, he's kind of funny.

"So, where did you live before here?"

"Well, I grew up in Jersey City and moved here when I was in elementary school. Since then, I've lived in California and Alaska, too."

"Alaska...you ever hear of Alaska Men magazine?" I asked.

"No. What's that?" He looked at me like I was up to something and I had to suppress my grin.

"So, there's a shortage of ladies up there, right? Guys advertise to get women to move there. The pictures are all really rugged. Like, 'Hi, I'm Steve. I like to chop things with my axe.' I saw a copy once and thought it was outstanding."

"Well, I can assure you I have never advertised in there."

"Not an axe man?" I asked, feigning disappointment.

He laughed. "No, I don't own an axe. Just note here that this would also disqualify me as an axe murderer. You know, in case that was a concern of yours."

"Duly noted, counselor."

I liked this guy.

"Would now also be good time to tell you you're my first blind date?" He asked.

"Seriously?"

He looked around conspiratorially before leaning in and whispering, "How am I doing?"

"In my learned opinion, I would say quite well, indeed," I whispered back.

Okay. I *really* liked this guy.

"So, wait—" I cut him off about an hour into our conversation, after learning he was seven years older than me, "when you were learning to drive, I was learning to spell."

"I prefer to think of it more like when I was finishing grad school you were starting college."

"That doesn't sound much better."

"It doesn't bother me. Does it bother you?"

"Less than I thought it would."

We kept talking well past the time our cups ran dry. Eventually, the café staff started flipping chairs onto the tables, a clear signal for us to get the heck out. It was past 11 p.m. We had closed down the joint.

But neither of us wanted to stop talking, so we took the 15 minutes and three jug handles back to his place.

We hung out into the small hours.

We've been hanging out ever since.

Hospital: Emergency Room

The doctor's business card felt flimsy in my hand.

The image of a pastel stethoscope circled the text like a lasso. Something about it bothered me. Something about *her* bothered me.

The emergency room had called her in for a consultation. She was a gastroenterologist, and based on the information on her card, this wasn't her usual hospital.

The staff at *this* hospital has a reputation for being personable. We knew that both from our past experience and the multiple awards for patient-centered care prominently on display.

It was clear this doctor's name would never make it onto one of those plaques. We waited for six hours, and she was to be the grand finale of our visit. I was eager for her to shed some light on what the problem was, prescribe some meds and then send us home. Instead, she skipped a greeting, handed me her obnoxious card, and flipped through Jim's chart in silence.

"You have cirrhosis," she announced curtly, breaking the silence.

"What?" Jim asked. "How?"

She pulled a copy of the ultrasound out of her folder and held it out to Jim. I leaned over the bed rail so I could view it, too.

"There are these nodules all around the liver. Didn't your primary care doctor show these to you?" There was something accusatory in her voice.

"Not exactly," Jim responded, more patient than I could have in that moment. "He said something about 'possible cirrhosis' and didn't share many details beyond that. He referred me to a specialist."

The doctor nodded. "Did you go see that specialist?"

"We tried to make an appointment," I chimed in.

"Tried?" The doctor said, looking down her nose at me skeptically. *Accuse much?*

"What my wife means to say is I booked an appointment and there is a wait of several weeks."

This seemed to mollify her.

"But, what does all this mean?"

"Oh. Your liver is severely compromised."

"But...how did this happen?"

She gave him a look that clearly said, *Oh, you so totally know how this happened.*

That was it. I loathed her with the fire and passion of a thousand suns. Jim and I simultaneously gave her the universal face for, "*And, your answer now, please?*"

She caved into our stares with a sigh. "Well, it is typically the result of long-term abuse—when people poison their liver with toxic substances."

"But Jim doesn't drink." She stared me down until I added, "Much. He doesn't drink much."

"I'm a lightweight," Jim said, trying to lighten the mood.

It was true. Jim liked drinks of the sugary, frozen, fruit-accented, umbrella-bedecked variety. He would have one, get a little happy, and then call it a night. Jim enjoyed the taste of booze more than the experience of booze. I had danced on enough tables to appreciate liquor's non-taste-related attributes.

"Seriously," I said. "This diagnosis makes no sense."

Jim went straight to business, "What does this mean for me—for my care?"

"Well, the first thing we're going to do is get all the fluid out of you." She began. Jim looked visibly relieved at that. "Then we're going to send it out for testing to see if you have an infection. If you do, we will treat it."

"So, once the infection clears, the liver will improve?" I asked.

"No, the liver is gone."

Jim and I looked at her like she was speaking gibberish. "What does that mean?"

"Cirrhosis means the liver is severely scarred."

Still struggling to comprehend what we were hearing, we asked her to repeat herself.

"The scarring means it's gone. Done. Barely functional. You must maximize the function you have left."

"And how much is that?"

"Probably only a few percent. I need to check his MELD." She began flipping through Jim's chart.

"Melt?" I asked.

The doctor seemed exasperated as she corrected me. "Meld. M-E-L-D. It's a score doctors use for liver function."

Jim had gone silent, but I had one more question. "Will he be admitted?"

"Yes. Let me get that abdominal tap started." She walked away.

I glared at her as she left the room. What did she really know, anyway? She didn't know Jim. She didn't know him at all. Who was she to imply he was a drug-addled, promiscuous boozer? Screw her and her crappy business card, too.

Jim and I said little to each other. In the absence of solid information, we both knew all we would have for each other was platitudes. After a few minutes, a hospital team member arrived to wheel Jim to his abdominal tap. I tried to follow along, but Jim held up his hand. "Why don't you stick around here and make some calls."

I did what he asked. I started by calling my parents. I also reached out to my best friend Reagan, in case she had to be on cat duty. The calls went fast, mostly because I had little to say. There were still too many unknowns. Plus, I didn't want to mention the word *cirrhosis*. The doctor's borderline-sarcasm attested to the fact that people jump to conclusions when they hear that swell diagnosis.

I just wasn't ready to deal with other people's reactions. I was still processing my own. I settled into the guest chair next to Jim's

Emergency Room bed and prepared for another long wait. After logging in to the hospital's Wi-Fi, I and searched: "MELD and liver."

The first result stated: *"MELD stands for Model for End Stage Liver Disease."*

Wait. What now? I paused for a moment, took a deep breath, and then typed: "MELD and death."

A chart filled my screen:

3-Month Mortality Based on MELD Scores:
Mortality Probability
MELD 40 71.3% mortality
MELD 30-39 52.6% mortality
MELD 20-29 19.6% mortality
MELD 10-19 6.0% mortality

We didn't know his score yet, but if this was true, there was at *least* a 6% chance Jim would die in the next 90 days.

My shaky fingers flew across my phone as I typed: "How do you reduce MELD score?"

Links send me to pages that were a little more wordy, and a lot more medical, but all roads lead to one answer:

Liver transplant.

Hospital: Jim's Room, Five Days Later

There had been a lot of activity and few answers.

Jim was on intravenous medication to fight the infection in his belly. He was also receiving several therapeutic taps to remove the fluid collecting in his abdomen. I've been to my share of frat picnics and know my way around a beer keg. After watching the procedure done on Jim, I can confirm the two processes are not dissimilar.

The World's Most Unpleasant Gastroenterologist did a daily drive-by to check on Jim's progress. She and the team were competent when it came to taking care of Jim's immediate problem — infection.

However, at no point during Jim's stay did anyone address the lingering threat — cirrhosis. As I heard the word "discharge" being bandied about, finding someone to manage Jim's condition in an ongoing capacity became that much more pressing.

My cell phone rang. I looked at the display. Word about Jim's condition was spreading amongst our friends, so I had been fielding phone calls and texts for the past few days.

"It's Mitch." I told Jim, "I'm going to step out to take this."

To save time updating everyone, I had started a Facebook group to post updates on Jim's health. Mitch and his wife, Lisa, were mutual friends. In that moment, I realized the first they heard of his condition was via that group invite. I clearly had explaining to do.

"The timing was terrible," I told Mitch. "Jim had been trying to get in to see a local gastroenterologist. He's supposed to be great. Jim made an appointment with the guy, but it was about two months out."

"What's the name of the doctor?"

"Kenney, I think. Dr. Kenney."

I heard Mitch laugh, "Steve Kenney?"

"I think that's it." My pulse quickened.

"Next town over, right?"

"Yeah."

"Let me call you right back."

Mitch is that friend who would call a car company CEO to make the company pay for new brakes not covered by the warranty because, well...Mitch thinks they should have been. Mitch is never rude, but he can be single-minded and assertive *in extremis.*

I pictured Mitch driving over to the doctor's office, slamming his hands on the registration desk, and demanding Dr. Kenney see my ailing husband. I envisioned picket signs and #SaveJim leaflets. I wasn't sure how far he would take it, and I really didn't want to add *bail Mitch out of jail* to my growing to-do list. I was about to hit redial to tell him to stop doing whatever he planned on doing when my phone rang. He was calling me back.

"Dr. Kenney will be at the hospital in about two hours," Mitch said, glee in his voice.

It was a Saturday. One doesn't just summon a doctor to a hospital on a Saturday. "Today?" I asked, a hint of suspicion and concern in my voice. "In two hours?"

"That's how long it will take for his kids to finish their game."

Okay. This sounds like stalking. "What. Did. You. Do?"

"I texted him and asked him to come see you after the kids' game was over."

It turned out Mitch and Lisa were good friends with Dr. Kenney and his wife.

That was when I learned that I had already met Dr. Kenney several months earlier. Mitch and Lisa throw an epic party every year, which involves them turning the entire first floor of their house into a karaoke bar. They don't just plug a microphone into big screen TV. They build a stage in their basketball court-sized foyer and roll out a professional sound system and theatrical lighting.

It was now my hope that the good doctor appreciated my a-little-more-than-tipsy rendition of *Pour Some Sugar on Me.*

Hospital: Jim's Room, Exactly One Hour and 45 Minutes Later

After the requisite jokes about wishing we'd seen each other under better circumstances and his tactful non-mention of Def Leppard, Dr. Kenney got down to business.

He reiterated a lot of what we'd already learned — Jim's health had become a serious issue and his liver was failing. He also helped us fill in a lot of our knowledge gaps.

At that point, all we had been told was that excessive drinking and drug abuse cause liver damage. This is true, but other things can also cause *liver* damage. Our surly gastroenterologist had left that part out.

Another potential culprit is hepatitis, a virus which causes liver inflammation and can lead to scarring. You can sometimes get Hepatitis A from contaminated food. The most common way for the various flavors of Hepatitis — A, B, or C — to pass from one person to another, however, is through blood and other bodily fluids. Think: Unprotected sex and needle sharing.

Jim and I were big on unfiltered conversations. We had shared our life stories with each other years ago. I didn't expect that he'd edited out long chapters featuring hookers and heroin, but if that was a factor here, the doctor needed to know, and I offered to leave the room so they could speak privately. Jim declined and then tested negative for Hepatitis.

They had ruled pretty much every vice out.

The next usual suspect was liver cancer, but Dr. Kenney told us of that possibility in the same breath with which he informed us they'd ruled that out in Jim's case.

Dr. Kenney was flipping through a small stack of paperwork as he talked to us. What the in-hospital gastroenterologist lacked in bedside manner, it turned out she made up for in thoroughness. She had commissioned every test result and report Dr. Kenney was now reading.

"My theory is that the most likely culprit is NASH," he finally said, setting aside the documents.

"As in Crosby, Stills and...?" I joked.

"Spelling-wise? Yes. As to the cause? No. NASH stands for *nonalcoholic steatohepatitis* and falls under the broader category of *nonalcoholic fatty liver disease* (NAFLD)."

People with NAFLD have an accumulation of fat in their liver, but no accompanying symptoms. Fatty liver most often presents itself in routine blood tests as elevated alanine aminotransferase (ALT) and aspartate aminotransferase (AST) levels. When a doctor sees these results, he or she will typically send the patient for an imaging scan of the liver.

Plenty of people have a fatty liver. There are over three-million cases in the United States per year — roughly one out of every hundred people. Risk factors include obesity, type-2 diabetes, and those with an underlying metabolic syndrome.

While NAFLD is not necessarily a *good* thing, it is not a terrible thing either. A fatty liver is a chronic condition that can be managed, or even completely reversed, by changes in diet and lifestyle. Over 80% of people with a fatty liver do not develop any serious problems. But for some people — that other 20% — a fatty liver can take a sinister turn. The fat in the liver causes inflammation, which causes cell damage. This cell damage then creates scar tissue. This is when

NAFLD turns to NASH. For some people with NASH, the scarred tissue overtakes the remaining healthy liver tissue.

Hello, cirrhosis!

The challenge with NASH is there is no blinking neon sign saying: *Serious Liver Problem Here.* It just quietly happens in the background.

In Jim's case, there were vague signs of problems, but nothing that raised major red flags. Jim had type-2 diabetes, but we thought that a byproduct of his recent weight gain. I figured depression, triggered by his mom's passing, caused him to put on a few pounds.

Dr. Kenney informed us the weight gain is because of fluid collection. As Jim's liver was totally crapping out, fluids were building up in his abdomen — a condition called *ascites.* What I'd read as sadness-induced jelly belly was something else entirely.

Jim had also gotten an odd blood test about two years prior. He spent roughly 24 months working as a civilian reconstruction specialist in Iraq. He loved his work there and was trying to extend his contract and get a gig with the U.S. State Department. In a surprise twist, they passed on Jim because he failed the medical examination because of a higher-than-normal bilirubin score.

When Jim came home, he went to a specialist who'd seen nothing of consequence in Jim's health. Yes, Jim had a fatty liver, but there was no scarring or anything to cause alarm. The doctor basically said, "Welcome back to the United States. Eat more salad." A second opinion confirmed the same.

There was no tidy answer to explain why this had happened. It just happened. Now Jim and I had to deal with our new normal. Jim had less than 10% liver function, and this function would only get worse.

Dr. Kenney kindly offered to serve as Jim's doctor in the short-term, but strongly urged us to get an appointment with a team specializing in transplants.

There was a grand total of one hospital in New Jersey which did this.

Seven Years Ago

With me just about to pass the thirty-year mark, we decided it was time to have kids.

Things started out quite promising. Very shortly after we threw away the birth control pills, a pee stick test revealed two faint lines. We went through the entire cycle of emotions — surprise, disbelief, amazement, excitement, fear of doing an awful job and the hope we'd do a magnificent job and prove ourselves wrong.

We were in the starting-to-tell-people stage when I felt a stitch in my side while driving to work. The pain got progressively worse. I called my OBGYN from my desk phone and was told to come in to the office right away. After an in-office ultrasound, they rerouted me to the hospital. My day ended on the operating table. Ectopic pregnancy.

What followed was a five-year fertility odyssey. We completely lived our lives according to fertility specialist recommendations. No heated seats. No hot tubs. No drinking. Inject myself in the morning; take oral meds later. Get blood drawn. Have sex on a schedule. Pee on a stick. Get disappointed. Cry my eyes out. Rinse and repeat.

Every period felt like a giant failure.

We ratcheted up our efforts. I got injected with dye and had a few more doctor's visits. Jim had bodily fluids sent to labs, and we progressed to Intrauterine Insemination (IUI).

If you are unfamiliar with the process, this is how it works: Guy drops off his *sperm*, lady shows up two hours later to get injected with said sperm. This *all felt a bit impersonal.* So, Jim and I made a date of it. I accompanied him to the drop off. We then went to a nearby diner for the two-hour wait. We thought a hearty breakfast of bacon would entice our would-be offspring to hang around for a while. *There will be more of this in your future, zygote!* When we returned to the doctor, Jim watched daytime television in the lobby while they escorted me to a room in the back, to make me a mom.

Our breakfast-as-encouragement strategy did not yield the hoped-for results.

It appeared all of our friends and family members were having children. They frequently asked me, "So, are you and Jim thinking about having kids?"

I wanted to answer, "Why yes. I think about it often. It's all-consuming, actually. We have built the entirety of our lives together around the fruitless pursuit of offspring. I am barely holding it together at this point. Thanks so much for asking!"

What came out instead was, "Well... " *knowing giggle*, "if it happens, it happens!"

It would have been great to point to a reason, but there was none. We had unexplained infertility. It just...was.

In the professional realm of infertility treatment, there is always someone who will offer you hope at the right price. Jim and I had reached the "*spending the equivalent of a college education to do the work of God*" point in our infertility odyssey when we called it quits.

Jim and I were always more practical than spiritual. All signs pointed to parenthood being a no go. Our decision to stop didn't result from a bone-deep belief that the universe had something different and special planned for us, but instead from a shared understanding that we just didn't want to be miserable anymore.

A psychologist would probably have told us we were experiencing a period of grief. But, after already investing thousands of dollars on our loins, we didn't want to add therapy bills on top of that. Instead, we developed our own coping mechanisms.

I reconsidered my religious beliefs. If I did everything right, was a good person, kind to pets, and paid my taxes — why did God feel I wasn't good enough? Why did thieves and addicts and all-around-bad-people get to be so incredibly fertile and I just wasn't?

I went full-tilt atheist.

Jim took things another direction, casually saying one night over dinner:

"I think I'd like to go work in Iraq."

Points to him for creativity.

For the next two years, that's what he did. He applied for and received a provincial reconstruction job in Baghdad. I thought this was an unusual choice for a municipal attorney-turned-lobbyist with a thirst for adventure until I learned more about the gig.

Following the Iraq War, the governance situation needed work. Iraq had a national government (that was getting a post-Saddam overhaul). What Iraq did not have was a formal government structure on a local level - things like state, county, and municipal government. For the citizens of Iraq, this meant a lack of shared civic services — such as fire departments, schools, and hospitals.

Jim's job was to encourage cooperation between factions, often with very divergent views, through a variety of projects intended to establish a regional government structure while building bringing sustainable services to the people of Iraq.

The work was interesting, exhausting, and sometimes dangerous, and Jim absolutely loved it.

Our relationship found its way through our frequent Skype calls and *meet in the middle somewhere* vacations. We travelled to Paris, Amsterdam — even hot and sunny Vegas (my choice, not Jim's).

It was nice not to have every conversation be about making babies. We were each doing our own thing, and we were enjoying each other, doing each other's own thing.

While Jim was overseas, I was navigating my career in the U.S. I made a job change to a start-up and took on DIY improvements to the house.

It was an unusual arrangement to be sure, but somehow, it worked for us.

The two years flew by and he asked if I would mind him staying abroad for a third. I figured, why not? He would do that for one more year and then we could figure out our future. The money was good. We were both happy. We also had some very cool Christmas cards to show for it. The one showing a smiling Jim in front of Saddam's former palace was a particular favorite.

However, because of his medical examination, the United States Department of State declined to make him an offer. Jim had no choice but to come home.

We didn't dwell on this news because, just as all this was unfolding, Jim's mother got sick.

Jim's mom, Ellie, had persistent infections keeping her in and out of the hospital. It was a regular cycle — hospital, rehabilitation center, home. Repeat this every two weeks for a year. Every time it happened, she lost a little more of her spark. I had been her primary caregiver during the first part of Jim's working abroad until she later re-located south where Jim's sister then took on that role. Despite getting the best of care, Ellie just wasn't improving. By the time she passed away, surrounded by family in the hospital, she ready to go.

Jim put off his job search to care for his mom and then to settle her affairs. During this time, Jim started complaining of fatigue. He also gained a lot of weight. He started pulling away and turning in to himself.

"Jim, are you all right?" I asked him one morning when he seemed especially down.

"Getting by," he reassured me with a half smile. "Just tired."

"Maybe therapy," I said tentatively. He nixed the idea every time I brought it up. "You've just been through so much..."

"No." He said firmly. "No therapy."

"Honey, you must do something."

"I'm going to see the doctor next week to see what's going on."

"Okay. That's good. That's really good."

Facebook Group
Jim's Liver Party
June 12

TJ: "Looks like Jim is getting out of the hospital today (fingers crossed!) or tomorrow. He is in excellent hands (Dr. Kenney) now and will soon go to a liver specialist familiar with transplants. In the meantime, the plan is no booze (duh), meds (for infection) and keeping a very careful eye on his fluids. (Basically, he has to weigh himself daily, making sure what he is putting in is coming out, etc. We want to do whatever possible to make sure he doesn't need draining!) He is also on a very, very low-sodium diet so I can no longer continue my classy practice of putting the box of Morton's salt out on the table every time we eat."

CHAPTER 2: MID JUNE

Our House, Central NJ

Dr. Kenney strongly recommended we take Jim to a liver specialist familiar with transplants. However, he couldn't actually recommend or refer us to one, because none of his patients had ever been sick enough to need a transplant. Under different circumstances, I would have saluted Dr. Kenney on his excellent doctoring. But, as it stood now, I had a husband with a time bomb of a liver and needed to find another doctor STAT.

After a good bit of Internet sleuthing and phone calls, I identified the Liver Center of NJ, which had the distinction of being the only liver transplant center in the state. This made the choice pretty easy.

I called to make an appointment for Jim, the big day a little over a month away.

In the meantime, Jim had some lifestyle changes to make. Dr. Kenney gave Jim his marching orders:

1. Continue to take medicine to treat the infection. This (we hoped) would keep Jim from making a repeat appearance at the hospital.
2. Stop drinking booze. This surprised absolutely no one. Jim expressed disappointment when he remembered his last drink had been a semi-warm wine cooler at a friend's gathering.
3. Limit salt intake to a little over 1,500 milligrams a day, roughly the equivalent of a half teaspoon.

They also shared all of this information in a conspicuously cheerful hospital discharge packet.

There were detailed instructions about medication. There was a list of adverse symptoms and advice to call if/when we discovered any of them. There were encouraging words to the patient about self-care. There was also a photocopied-to-within-an-inch-of-its-life nutritional pamphlet. Said pamphlet featured a picture of a smiling nurse handing a maniacally joyful octogenarian a half-peeled banana. Below the primary goal (in this case, reducing sodium intake), it provided lists of suggested foods, along with helpful hints such as, "Apples and carrots are a delicious snack for those looking to manage their salt."

Jim already excelled at banana peeling and, as enjoyable as they could be, he couldn't live on apples and carrots alone. I needed more guidance. Bring on the Internet.

Limiting salt to 1,500 — 2,000 milligrams a day considered part of the *healthy-heart diet*. It is the salt-level guideline given to patients with hypertension.

Makes sense. A healthy heart is good, right? I told myself.

Step One: Throw out the bag of salted pretzels I'm currently eating while browsing the Internet.

Step Two: Decide to make this a fun team project.

I pictured Jim and I holding hands while noshing on unsalted crackers smeared with grape jelly. *Our situation has the potential to be both nutritious and romantic.*

Step Three: Figure out how to make this work.

In order to do that, we need to talk about salt.

Salted bagels. Salting the driveway. Salt-N-Pepa. We live in a world of sodium chloride, and I was a lifelong fan.

Sea. Kosher. Pink. Volcanic. I loved it all.

Friends had even suggested I invest in a deer salt lick for my own snacking. The idea wasn't out of the realm of reason. Let me put it this way: I salt *canned* soup.

The primary reason I got to enjoy this privilege was that I was blessed with an undeservedly low resting blood pressure. My heart was a sailor swimming in a salty sea of blood brine.

But my mate could no longer indulge. Time for some adjustments.

Jim was still feeling pretty wretched, so the shopping, cooking and, dare I say, imagination all fell to me.

I begin with the easy wins of salt avoidance:

Processed foods are the biggest salt offenders, think: frozen meals, cold cuts, hot dogs, ham, soy sauce, just about anything in a can, and anything with a flavor packet. Toodle-oo tuna fish. Bye-bye bacon, and deli turkey, packages of cheesy rice, and all their delicious equivalents.

To give you a sense of scope — a pouch of powdered Noodle Soup is roughly an entire day's worth of salt.

Lesser-known salt offenders include things like bread, crackers, cheese, pickles, peanut butter, salad dressing, ketchup, mustard, and barbeque sauce.

Now, here's where it gets difficult. Sneaky offenders include butter, fish (because it's from the salty sea), meat (because sometimes it's brined), baking soda, and instant pudding.

Let's also factor in personal preferences. Jim does not like vegetables that taste *wet*, including (but not limited to): tomatoes, zucchini, squash, and sliced-too-thick eggplant.

I found some empty boxes, went through the pantry and removed every item Jim could no longer eat. On the upside, I could finally see the back wall of our pantry. On the downside, all that remained was a bag of rice and a dusty jar of apple butter.

Looking at our now-bare larder, I considered my options.

Jim was still weak from his time in the hospital and slow moving because of fluid retention. He wasn't able to stand or walk for long periods of time. Spending an hour or more in the kitchen chopping and sauteing was a no-go for him. What complicated matters was that I traveled nearly 90% of the time for work. I couldn't be around consistently to shop for and prepare fresh meals.

So, the goal was for everything in the house to be something Jim could get from the fridge/freezer/cabinet, to the microwave, and then to the coffee table (his current dining space of choice) in fewer than 10 minutes.

It was time to strategize. In the business realm, when you lack sufficient expertise and resources to tackle a problem, your best option is to outsource.

I looked into several places that promised healthy, chef-prepared meals of the heat-and-eat variety. I did a deep dive into the menus and nutritional information and quickly discovered there weren't many options for liver patients. Outsourcing was off the table.

My next thought was to look at my supply chain. I figured there had to be other people out there with Jim's dietary restrictions who were enterprising enough to set up shop. I found an online store for heart patients which offered pantry staples with really low or no salt. Huzzah! A case of no-salt sloppy joe mix and about 30 other no-sodium delicacies were on their way to our doorstep.

While I could now avoid going full Amish on this — a la homemade ketchup making — I would still need to cook. The new schedule involved me strapping on an apron every Saturday morning and doing an all-day cooking marathon to make and freeze a week's worth of food. I was on my way to becoming the next celebrity chef for the cirrhosis set.

I went online and binge-shopped for cookbooks with titles like *Cooking Without a Grain of Salt* and *Cooking Without: All Recipes Free from Added Gluten, Sugar, Dairy, Yeast, Salt and Saturated Fat*. I even got very creative (after three glasses of wine on a Friday night) and created a compendium of recipes called *Jim's Yum Book*. When I showed its namesake the fruit of my scissored labors, Jim seemed unimpressed. I think perhaps this was because it didn't include a recipe for soy-glazed bacon.

The first recipe I tried was ginger chicken lettuce wraps with a homemade plum sauce. By the time I served our meal, with great flourish, out on our back deck, I had already spent four hours cooking. Drenched in sweat, I had only two small freezer containers of food to show for all my efforts. The food was tasty, but my model was unsustainable. I needed to try simpler fare.

Thus, the standard Condon family meal was born. It looked a little something like this: chicken breast liberally sprinkled in no-salt seasoning, a side of rice accented with a pat of unsalted butter and some vegetables on the side, accented with a bit more unsalted butter. Dessert was something that wasn't pudding.

Mrs. Dash no-salt seasoning became my go-to, especially because it came in many varieties. You want lemon-pepper chicken? Check. You want that chicken to taste like an herb garden? No problem. You feeling a little zesty? Well, Mrs. Dash makes Mexican-themed sprinklings. Ole!

While I could help Jim meet his nutritional needs, this transition to a new normal was not entirely smooth.

Jim liked grocery shopping and took great pride in it. He is a committed couponer and has this freaky ability where he can remember exactly how much or how many remain in any bottle or box and can predict exactly when we'd need another. Over the years of our marriage, I'd learned a question like, "Did you notice you're eating more cheddar?" was not Jim's way of saying, "Lay off the cheese, fatty!" Rather, it was him cataloging food preferences and doing some secret math in his head to make sure we never ran out of anything we liked. Everyone's favorites needed to be on hand at all times. Jim's calculation of projected pickle consumption was just another way of saying, "I love you."

For the time being, Jim couldn't be the family's shopper. This irked him.

He could also no longer eat what he liked. This irked him, too.

For the first time in his life, a medical condition prevented him from doing the everyday things virtually all of us take for granted. Jim had to process all the news about his declining health, while also feeling an acute loss of control.

Emotions are interesting things. You may try to work through things and see the bright side. But those emotions? They don't just go away. They're still there. They can come out in unexpected ways. Jim was no exception. Soon after his diagnosis and return home, dinner conversations went a lot like this one:

"How much salt is in this?"

"Roughly 50 milligrams."

"What do you mean roughly?"

"It depends on the size of the piece you are eating. It would fall between 45-55. I estimated 50."

"Are you sure?"

"Yeah. I can hand you the package." I put down my fork, walked to the counter and picked up the package. Handing it to Jim, I resumed eating.

"I will need a scale, too." He stared at me impatiently. I put down my fork, walked to the counter and picked up the food scale, setting it in front of him before trying to go back to my meal. Jim took his food and put it on the scale.

"You should probably put down a paper towel first. I can get that for you."

I got halfway out of my seat before he responded. "That will affect the weight."

"Okay." I took a single bite as he continued to mess with the scale.

"What about the rice?"

"You mean the salt count on the rice?"

"Yes."

"Figure on 3 mg. You have about a cup-and-a-half there."

"About?"

"You have exactly a cup and a half there. I measured."

"Did you measure dry or cooked?"

I put down my fork.

"Cooked. You have a cup and a half of cooked rice on your plate."

"But there's butter on it."

"Yes. There is unsalted butter on it."

"Did you measure it with or without the butter on it?"

"What?"

"Because it would stick together and maybe measure out differently."

Now picture this conversation happening every single day, multiple times a day, with every single piece of food Jim put in his mouth.

"Can you hand me the applesauce package? I want to check the salt."

"Roughly 2mg. A cup is 5mg. Those servings are pretty tiny. So, I would say 2-3mg."

"I just want to check the package."

"Okay. Fine."

I handed him the package, and he looked it over. "You were right. I just wanted to make sure, you know? There's this other brand that might have less salt. Can you get that next time?"

"Sure. Happy to."

"When are you going to the store again?"

"Day after tomorrow, I think."

"We might run out sooner than that."

"Of what?"

"Of applesauce."

"You have two six-packs here. Do you really think you'll eat your way through all that applesauce?"

"I might."

"You have my solemn promise. If you run out of applesauce, I will immediately go out and buy replacement applesauce."

"Thanks. You know, I'm not trying to be annoying here."

"I know, I know."

"I just want to make sure there's something I can eat that won't blow my salt count."

I took a deep breath and reflected on the refrigerator, freezer and cabinets I had spent hours filling with home-cooked and nutritionally vetted foods compliant with Jim's unique dietary requirements and taste preferences. I then considered poking him repeatedly with my fork. Instead, I went with...

"I know. I totally get that."

That night, we watched TV together.

"I can't believe how much salt they're using in that! The chef should really lighten up."

Well, cooking shows are out.

"That street food looks amazing. I just wish they would use less soy sauce."

Okay. Travel shows are also out.

I was now specifically reading program descriptions to make sure no one was chewing on an episode.

This was our existence for a few weeks. Make blandish food. Eat blandish food. Discuss salt content of blandish food. Repeat.

Only a few people knew the extent of Jim's illness. He and I avoided the topic because, frankly, it was a bummer. We used *Jim's Liver Party* on Facebook to share occasional medical updates with family and close friends, but we tried to keep it as light as possible. People go to Facebook to see cat memes and argue about politics — not to get blow-by-blows of someone's illness. If we got an invitation from a friend to do something, we would just politely decline.

Jim's health seemed to be on an upswing now that doctors and medicine managed the infection. So, when Mitch and Lisa asked us to go out, we made the choice to accept. We hadn't had a night out in ages. Seeing friends would be nice.

Now Mitch likes food — a lot. He is always on the quest to find the best this or that. He and Lisa had raved about this local pizza place and suggested we go there.

I was about to request we go to a different place because of Jim's circumstances, but Jim stopped me. He had eaten nothing but hospital food and home-cooked meals in weeks. He had a hankering for some real pizza. (Being from New Jersey, this is not a surprise.) With some planning and preparation, he could make a meal out doable. We couldn't eat at home forever. He didn't have to say goodbye to restaurants forever. This was a good trial run.

The night before, and the morning of, Jim did everything he could not to ingest so much as a single atom of salt. He wanted to reserve all of his salt intake for pizza time.

When we arrived at the appointed time, Mitch poured over the menu, narrating all the choices.

"Should we get sausage? Pepperoni? Meatballs? Maybe the BBQ chicken? There's even one that has Caesar dressing on it."

Jim had studied the menu online a few days in advance and realized pretty quickly he had limited options. All "exotics" were out for him. When we all sat at the table together, I made a brief mention of Jim's "special diet" and said he would probably do his own ordering. I assumed Jim's plan was to stick to plain pizza — one or two slices, depending on the size.

I didn't expect Jim to ask Mitch and Lisa about the ingredients. While Mitch and Lisa knew the owner of the place, they didn't work in the kitchen. As Jim's questions got more specific, I got more uncomfortable.

"What is in the crust? Is the cheese shredded or homemade? If they use chicken, what do they season it with? How big are the meatballs?"

Mitch, unable to answer the questions, offered to introduce us to the owner who had recently become a friend of his and Lisa's.

"Oh, I don't want to bother the guy," I said.

"No, he'll be happy to come out and say hi," Mitch assured me.

The owner came over. After some pleasantries, Jim asked questions about the food. The owner seemed pleased Jim had taken such an interest. Jim's questions kept getting increasingly in-depth. About 10 minutes into the conversation, Jim asked this:

"So, is your sauce bottled or made here?"

In a New Jersey pizza place, this question is akin to, "Would you mind if I have sex with your mother?" I couldn't take it anymore, and when I get embarrassed, I go full polite — like southern cotillion polite. So I chimed in, "Honey, it's clearly made here! Look at those folks in the kitchen. Not a jar or can of sauce in sight. We are in for such a treat! Thank you so much for coming to speak with us today." As the owner walked away, I turned back to Jim. "Honey, how about this? Let's let Mitch and Lisa get what they want, and you can do your own order?"

Jim's face hardened. "I was trying to do that. I still had some more questions for that guy."

"I know, but he has a restaurant to run. You've already asked a lot of questions. How about..."

"You mean I'm not allowed to ask questions about what I put in my mouth?"

"Of course, you can ask questions. But there comes a time when you have to be practical."

"I WILL ORDER WHAT I WANT, WHEN I WANT!"

The place went quiet. All heads turned toward us.

In that very moment, we became the couple who yells at each other in public, at a pizza place, no less.

My face suddenly flamed. My heart thrummed erratically. I was about to blow. I needed to get away. "I need a minute." I said as politely as I could. I wiggled out of the booth and sprinted to the ladies' room in the back of the restaurant.

I rarely cry, but when I do, it is epic. We're talking keening, moaning accompanied by great heaving sobs. I am not a quiet crier, either. Or a neat crier.

I must have been loud enough to hear over the Little League pizza party taking place near the restrooms, because Lisa came in to check on me. Having never seen me cry before, she approached me with the extreme caution of a zookeeper treating an injured tiger.

"So, are you guys, like, doing...okay?"

I almost wanted to laugh. "No. No, we're not. We're not at all."

...Well, at least that's what I wanted to say. Instead, I mumbled something about it being "a weird day." I sponged my tears with wadded up paper towels.

It's not that she wouldn't have understood. She'd experienced a pretty serious illness herself a few years ago. She'd stayed strong throughout her ordeal but had also been very honest about the feelings and the general weirdness that came along with it. If I'd talked about our situation, Lisa would have understood. She also was the very textbook definition of a patient and sympathetic listener. The universe could not have sent me better bathroom company right now.

But I couldn't bring myself to share. I could barely process my feelings, let alone give voice to them. This wasn't about the pizza. Frankly, it wasn't even about Jim's unscrupulous attention to food detail. Even before his most recent issues, he had always been one of those guys who would ask at least five questions of the server. This was just a heightened version of normal.

I was mourning simplicity. Did we need to plan for every contingency now because the world could fall apart at any moment? Could a pizza ever just be a pizza anymore?

I headed for the door.

"You might need another minute," Lisa told me, as politely as possible. "How about I meet you at the table?"

When she left, I looked at myself in the mirror, red-faced and disheveled. No makeup bag in the world was going to fix this. As I listened to a disco version of *That's Amore* on the bathroom speakers, I did my best to wipe off the streaks of mascara.

When I returned to the table, the menus were gone. Jim and Mitch had ordered pizza for the table and the trio was was now talking about movies.

Jim, who has the rare gift of being immune to social discomforts, either failed to notice the bedraggled state of his wife sliding into the booth beside him or wisely ignored it. Instead, he grabbed my hand under the table and gave it a squeeze.

CHAPTER 3: JULY

City Hospital, Liver Center, Waiting Room

We were to meet with a hepatologist — a liver specialist — attached to the liver center. We were to bring all of Jim's medical records. We were to show up 15 minutes before our 10 a.m. appointment to allow for check-in time.

When we arrived at 9:31 a.m., it was a completely packed house. They probably meant for the waiting room to accommodate 30 people, yet somehow 50 squeezed in. Jim tried to find a place to sit while I got him sorted out at the front desk.

As I handed him the clipboard and stack of forms from the receptionist. He glanced around the room.

"So, this is what liver transplant looks like," he said. The room contained a cross section of people — the quite old to the quite young, every color, every ethnicity, and probably a good cross-section of faiths, too.

I'd thought this room would look like a pub at closing time, with some guy muttering to no one in particular, while sipping brown liquor out of a paper bag. This place seemed more dentist's office than neighborhood bar. It also had all the doctor's office staples — television playing daytime TV and magazines from every genre.

What struck me was how well people looked. Sure, they seemed a little subdued. I mean, no one was jumping on trampolines at a hepatologist's office. But it looked as if they *could*. Compared to these people, Jim looked like a sick guy. His color was off. His stomach bulged. He barely had the energy to shave. My concern-o-meter registered this.

As the minutes went by, we saw a steady stream of people go in and out.

Hours went by.

Patients in. Patients out.

There were now only six people left in the room. It was 1 p.m. We waited.

Nearing 3 p.m., Jim and I were the last two people in the room.

A cheerful, petite lady with a stack of papers and an enormous purse opened the door to the waiting room. She walked towards the exit, about to leave for the day. She startled a bit when she saw us.

"Oh, hello there! I didn't expect to see anyone. Who are you here to see today?"

"Dr. Attia."

"Do you have an appointment? May I have your name?"

"Condon. C-O-N-D-O-N, as in 'Nancy.'" Jim said.

"Like London with a 'C.'" I added.

"May I ask how long you have been waiting?"

Jim and I looked at each other. We were not sure how to answer. I dived on the grenade.

"Well, our appointment was at 10 a.m..."

"Oh my. Come in. Come in!"

She asked another member of the staff if they could get us settled and grab our paperwork.

After a brief wait, the door opened once more to reveal the same woman, only she had stashed her purse and paperwork and was now wearing a pristine lab coat. The name stitched into her coat read *Dr. Attia*.

She asked Jim to lie down on the small exam table. He was stiff from hours of sitting and his size made lying down on the small table difficult. Dr. Attia and I each grabbed hold of an arm and helped him to lay back.

Dr. Attia spent a goodly amount of time near his belly, but also examined his hands, legs and feet.

What I liked about her was she kept her focus on Jim — asking how he felt, asking him what hurt.

As she helped sit him up, the questions continued. Bit by bit, Jim started opening up. The conversation even went beyond the medical stuff. He talked about his mom's passing. He talked about his worry and stress. Dr. Attia listened with great focus and asked many follow-up questions.

"Okay," she said, "So, let's get medical. We measure the health of liver patients using something called a MELD score."

"Model for End-stage Liver Disease, right?" I responded, because I guess I needed to feel like a smarty-pants in that moment.

"Exactly right! Although, I would like it better if it had a different name."

I couldn't decide if I wanted to adopt this doctor or ask her to be my new best friend.

She then gave us the complete MELD score rundown.

Dr. Patrick Kamath of the Mayo Clinic originally developed the MELD scoring system. Today the United Network for Organ Sharing (UNOS) uses MELD as the objective measuring tool for prioritizing organ allocation.

MELD is made up of three different patient values: Serum bilirubin, Serum creatinine, and International Normalized Ratio for Prothrombin Time (INR).

Serum bilirubin or, to keep it simple, *bilirubin*, is the healthy byproduct made when red blood cells break down in the body. The liver makes that bilirubin water-soluble, which helps your body excrete it. (Have you ever wondered why your pee is yellow? Now you know!) Those with unhealthy livers cannot process bilirubin effectively, which means it collects in the body, unable to be effectively excreted. Therefore liver patients are lemon colored.

The body makes serum creatinine, or *creatinine* for short, when muscles break down — normal wear and tear type stuff. When creatinine hits the bloodstream, the kidneys process it. Kidneys sometimes wind up picking up the slack when the liver is breaking down. Overwhelmed kidneys present on a blood test as a high creatinine score.

International Normalized Ratio for Prothrombin Time (INR) is a measure of how well or poorly your blood clots. A normal INR is 1.0. Every 0.1 higher means your blood is getting thinner and takes longer to clot. In liver patients, this happens because the liver is no longer making sufficient proteins to help blood clot normally.

33

For the people who did well in math and/or science class, here's the calculation:

MELD(i) = 0.957 × ln(Cr) + 0.378 × ln(bilirubin) + 1.120 × ln(INR) + 0.643* (*See Medical Note for additional information on MELD scores.)

For the rest of us, there are several calculators online. There's even a MELD app.

"Right now, Jim has a MELD of 17," Dr. Attia concluded.

"Is that...bad?" Jim asked.

"I don't really like to think of it in those terms. What I will say is 15 or higher means you are a candidate for a transplant."

"How high can these scores go?"

"Up to 40."

"So, this would mean Jim is, like, the healthiest of the really sick people?" I asked in all earnestness.

Dr. Attia smiled, "Well, that's one way to put it! Now we need to focus on making him feel better. While you will eventually need a transplant, we may postpone it for a long time."

"So... are you saying there's...hope?"

"There is a lot to be hopeful for, Jim."

She then said she had to step out of the room for a second to get something. Before she did, she nudged the tissue box on the counter toward me. Jim had tears streaming down his face.

Facebook Group
Jim's Liver Party
August 23

Jim: "Good news, bad news. Good news is my blood tests show I'm not getting any worse. Bad news is I'm not getting any better, either. Good news is my doctor is now placing me on a transplant list. Bad news is that getting a transplant, while necessary, is really not a lot of fun. Decisions, decisions. Meanwhile, I am rapidly shedding the fluid I had been retaining thanks to my medications, so I've got that going for me."

CHAPTER 4: AUGUST/SEPTEMBER

Our House

Jim's health had largely gone from "hospital bad" to "well-managed terminal illness bad."

Dr. Attia and people in the liver community were refreshingly direct. Jim's condition was terminal. He needed a transplant to extend his life.

Prior to Jim's organ extravaganza, my experience with transplantation was pretty limited.

Most of it came from a book I'd read in elementary school called *Making Half Whole.*

It was a book about twins, one of whom needed a kidney transplant. Kelly, my elementary BFF from up the street, an identical twin herself, recommended it.

Kelly and I had already devoured *The Baby-Sitters Club books* and the age-inappropriate-but-totally-awesome *Sweet Valley High* series. This was a diversion from our usual fare, but Kelly's gave it a strong recommendation.

"I read this and think it's fantastic. I'd like you to read it, too, and then we can talk about it."

She handed me her copy.

I still have the book, so like to think Kelly gave it to me because somehow both she and the cosmos knew there would be a time in the future I would really need it. Though, the more likely scenario is that I am forgetful and a book hoarder.

In the book, one of the teenage twins suffers from kidney disease. The author got the symptoms right — constant nausea, occasional confusion, debilitating exhaustion. When you are a kid, you think any disease involving possible fainting must be both serious and fabulous. The sick sister spent most of the book either at the doctor's office, on dialysis treatment or in bed. The illness took such a physical toll on the twin that the two sisters stopped looking alike.

The healthy twin was balancing maturity with healthy rebellion. She fiercely loved her ailing sister, but she was also just trying to live her life. For example, her ill sister couldn't eat pretzels (salt, baby), but she *really* loved pretzels and stowed a bag away in the basement for secret snacking. When her ill sister was out of earshot of crinkling plastic and crunching, the healthy sister would share pretzels with the omnipotent narrator of the book and confess her fears and frustrations while they noshed.

At some point, the healthy sister learned how she could be the hero who saved her sister's life as a living donor. Her parents kept trying to convince her that she was too young to consider such weighty matters, but the healthy sister wouldn't let up.

Serious spoiler alert here — the parents relented, and the operation was a rousing success. In record time, the twin girls were beautiful, healthy and whole.

It's a book about caring, sacrifice, sisterhood and parents who don't read.

I can tell you this book was Mayo Clinic worthy compared to your average television drama. With respect to transplants, there were at least two things every depiction got wrong — time and transformation. Getting transplant-qualified takes time, and for most patients, time is something in short supply.

As Jim's condition became more well known, I fielded a lot more questions.

Mostly, I appreciated when people took an interest. Educating myself on the facts and disseminating good information gave me a feeling of confidence. I felt as if I was becoming fluent in a language I had only just learned. If book reading, Internet sleuthing and educating others was a superpower, I intended to be the Wonder Woman of liver transplants.

The problem was that people were, well, human. They didn't always want to hear facts. More often, they wanted to share their knowledge and experiences, even if the "knowledge" came from the aforementioned television programs. People are reflexively helpful. At least that was what I would tell myself whenever a kindly soul spent 30 minutes telling me how they felt about their really distant cousin's organ transplant. They peppered the stories with enough bad medical information to make Dr. Thomas Starzl — father of transplantation surgery — rise from the grave and drive them to the library.

When they'd insert a real whopper, I would tactfully respond with facts. I intended this to gently nudge them to the truth. Sometimes I was successful, sometimes I was not. For those "not" times, I'd think of my mother standing next to a smiling Zombie Starzl, reminding me it was our family credo to be unfailingly polite.

One of the most common things I would hear was: "The liver can grow back."

So, let me set the record straight. This is true...ish. A *healthy* liver can regenerate. In fact, it's the only visceral organ able to do so. You may even start with a small piece of a liver (about 25%) and it can grow into full size. Livers are the starfish of body parts.

Neat, huh?

Over time, however, an unhealthy liver may become scarred, rendering it unable to regenerate. Severe scarring of the liver is what's known as cirrhosis. For people with cirrhosis, the medical path forward is to keep as much liver function as possible, for as long as possible.

Eventually, the cirrhotic liver will begin to decompensate (i.e. totally crap out). Doctors classify this as End Stage Liver Disease. When a patient reaches this stage, and this is the important bit here, *a transplant is the only option to prolong your life.*

Still, there were those who remained steadfastly convinced Jim's liver would just grow back—much like the majestic lizard, flatworm, or sea cucumber. Surely all this time Jim and I spent engaging with doctors was just our wild shenanigans.

The next thing people seem fixated on was the idea of the potential donor: "Will he get to pick/meet/hang out with the donor?"

With livers, that would almost always be a no. With pretty much all other transplantable organs (except kidneys), that would be a hard no.

I had a colleague — a truly well-educated person, whom I respect beyond measure — once say, "My cousin once got to meet her heart donor."

It took me a few seconds to respond because I chose my next words very carefully. "Do you mean the actual donor — the actual, *living* person — who gave their heart to your cousin?"

"The heart donor, yes. Lots of hugs and a really nice video. It was a really moving experience for her. I can send you the YouTube link."

What I think my colleague meant is that his cousin had a personal meeting with the donor's family. I am certain this moment was as powerful and moving as my colleague described. But I would bet my savings account, my cats, and all of my own organs on the fact that my colleague's cousin did not meet her heart donor. That donor no longer walks this earth. That donor instead made a beautiful, lasting and *final* gift.

Perhaps one of the hardest conversations I had to have during this time was about why I wasn't fun anymore.

Illness is about the daily administration of survival; you don't have room in your life for the frivolous. Fun is just not really an option anymore. You don't know what movies are playing in the theater. You're not thinking about hosting a barbecue. You're not planning your next vacation. At least one of you can't have a drop to drink. You're living on bland food and borrowed time. So yeah, the result is that you're kinda bad at parties.

A friend of mine, Sheila, was going through a rough time as well. Her father was ill, and she was travelling back and forth to see him.

We first met years ago by discovering we had many things in common, foremost our boyfriend. He had been dating both of us and, when that came to light, we dumped him and instead became lifelong friends.

After college, Sheila and I maintained a close relationship, swapping letters, then emails, then texts. Then, at a certain point, we kept track of each other through our posts on Facebook. However, my Facebook presence was purely me logging on to post the occasional update to *Jim's Liver Party*. I didn't scroll and read other people's updates. I just didn't have the time. Regrettably, a lot of those updates were Sheila talking about her father, and I didn't see a word of it.

During the week, I was almost never home because of my work and travel schedule. On Saturdays and Sundays when I was home, I was catching up on all the chores I couldn't do during the week and getting Jim's food and meds set up for the week ahead.

Rather than unpack this whole myriad of issues to my girlfriend, I referred to my general state of being as *busy*. I was too *busy* to get together. I was too *busy* to spend much time on social media. I was too *busy* to call or send a, "Hey, how are you doing?" email.

Sheila had fairly recently moved from Massachusetts to New Jersey, to a town about an hour north of me. I think her expectation was that I'd be able to hang out more. But the length of the drive made it hard to just kind of pop in. Finally, however, she insisted we get together at a pizza place equidistant to our homes.

That was when, for 45 minutes, she called me out as an awful friend as mozzarella congealed on my plate. I hurt her. I hadn't made time to see her. I hadn't reached out to her, despite everything that was happening with her dad. She was mad.

Part of me felt terrible, but the other part of me wanted to point out that I simply didn't know because I was dealing with my own struggles.

Our time together ended with me making apologies and promising to be a better, more attentive friend. For a short time, I was. But it all felt like one more responsibility on a growing list of unwelcome commitments.

It wasn't until a while later that she learned of Jim's condition from a mutual friend. She emailed offering help. I politely but firmly refused.

She meant well, but I had grown hard. I'd convinced myself I was doing just fine managing alone. I thought her kindness came with strings. I didn't want to forget to say thank you. I didn't want to make a critical social misstep and be on the receiving end of another pizza lecture.

I came to think of other relationships differently, as well. During my brief return to Facebook so I could keep up with Sheila's posts, I started noticing increasingly more theatrical indignation in my news feed.

I saw posts of one acquaintance's trip to Disney with complaints, such as:

"We got served drinks by the pool and they weren't even cold."

"The Mickey ice pops seem a lot smaller than our last visit."

"Some other families keep hogging the picture spots. Do you really need five whole minutes to take a photo?"

Her posts sparked great sadness in me. There were many things about her experiences that were just so far out of reach for us—children, travel, doing something for the fun of it. But I didn't feel bad for us. I felt bad for her. How sad to go through life feeling angry and disappointed all the time. I clicked *Unfriend*. I guarantee she didn't miss me, either.

I developed an allergy to fortunate complainers—those to whom many things are given, but still they find fault in them all.

Things were bad now—genuinely and legitimately bad. But we didn't have to feel bad all the time. There had to be a way to make light of our hard times. Because if we could feel good when things were dreadful, it would track that we would feel incandescently happy when things got better.

"I've been thinking about it a lot," I said to Jim one evening early on. "We need a motto or something."

"Like a slogan?"

"Yeah, something like that. This is going to get hard, right?"

"That's what she said." Jim said with a devious look in his eyes.

Exasperated sigh. "Seriously, there are times this is going to suck."

"That's what sh—"

I raised my hand to silence him. "Just focus, okay? So much about this is going to be bad, so we need to make it as not-bad as possible.

We need to go full stupid on this. Take every opportunity to smile and laugh."

"So, what you are saying is, can we make this fun?"

"Kind of?"

Jim turned to the cat. "What do you think?" The cat purred in ecstasy from Jim's loving attention. "The cat has ruled. Full stupid it is."

Facebook Group
Jim's Liver Party
September 23rd

TJ: "Yesterday, we hoisted sparkling cider and Shirley Temple martinis to Jim on his birthday. Today, we're headed to University Hospital for the half-day liver extravaganza where we talk to the social worker, financial counselor and patient counselor. Then, after *just* a few more tests, our hope is Jim — fingers crossed — gets approved for the transplant list by Halloween."

Our House

Jim's birthday was subdued but nice. Our friend Reagan came over. We cooked a super low-salt meal and finished it with a Venetian Table-inspired selection of mini cupcakes. Reagan and I indulged in some bubbly while Jim enjoyed some bubbly of his own—my very finest Shirley Temple, served in a chilled martini glass.

Getting on *The List* is a process. It's something which takes time, typically a few months. It's like a months-long series of job interviews, but with needles. You also spend more time in the car and in waiting rooms than you ever thought possible.

One doctor's appointment invariably led to another with a different-but-related doctor. Even routine care had extra complications. A simple dental cleaning now required back-and-forth calls between his dentist and the liver center, and a trip to the pharmacy for pre-visit antibiotics.

Jim also became a Zen master of waiting-on-hold. He would typically devote two or more hours a day to managing the complicated administration of being ill. Insurance claims needed review. Statements required frequent updates.

There was a recurring issue whereby every third blood test the lab billed him close to $2,000. Jim got very good at ferreting out the issue, usually involving some type of mis-coding. He would slog through the four hours of calls and faxes necessary to resolve it.

Jim is deliberate in that way. Having worked for a time in municipal government, he has a healthy respect for administration and bureaucracy. Having worked for a time in a war zone, he also appreciated the convenience of handling things by phone without getting shot at.

Now, let's talk about the mythical *List*.

What it actually is, is a national database maintained by the *United Network of Organ Sharing* (UNOS). UNOS knows all the patients in the United States who are waiting for transplant. Not all of those on the list will receive a transplant, because it is sadly a matter of demand outpacing supply. When patients submit their quarterly, monthly, and weekly blood tests via their transplant center, this is where the information goes.

The anonymized information in the UNOS database is publicly available. With a loved one, if you know a few factors, such as their MELD score, blood type, transplant hospital and age, you can see how they're doing in the "stats" relative to other patients. Those who study economics love this database because it is one of a kind and breathtakingly accurate. It is also a daily measure of life and death, which sometimes feels unnervingly like fantasy football.

What's often confounding to organ transplant newbies is how long the kidney list is when compared to the other organs. If most people have two of them and only need one, why is the list of people waiting for kidney transplants so long?

It's because kidneys are difficult to match because of several compatibility factors. That is why kidney patients and their families need to leverage marketing and recruitment skills, urging everyone in their acquaintance — friends, co-workers, church mates, and dog sitters — to get tested for compatibility and possibly become a living donor. I've had the privilege of meeting many of these living donors. Some gave to family members. Some gave to neighbors. Some gave to absolute strangers. All are exceptional human beings.

In the United States, it is illegal to buy an organ, so the expectation is that these donations are completely altruistic. That's why that urban myth about, "I woke up in a tub of ice" should no longer strike fear in the heart of an American. No surgeon in her right mind is going to go, "And this kidney came from where, now? Some dude in a bathtub? Well, hand me that scalpel, then!"

Livers are another story. While it is medically possible today to take a portion of a liver from a living donor and implant it in a waiting transplant patient, this practice is still rare. Most livers today come from a deceased donor. The donor is a person who registered their interest in donating their organs or whose family has made that decision on the donor's behalf.

What is important to understand is that not everyone who wishes to donate can actually do so — only approximately 1% of organ donors can give the gift of life. Only the organs of people who die in a hospital on a ventilator are suitable for transplant. The patient's doctors and nurses can't start a discussion about organ donation; the job of those doctors and nurses is to save the life of a patient. Rather, after the patient has experienced brain death, an Organ Procurement Organization (OPO) may start a discussion about donation. A qualified counselor from the OPO will talk to the family about how their loved one can help others live on.

Now imagine the emotions this family is going through. They are losing someone unbelievably precious to them — a father, mother, daughter, son — and they are being asked to prolong the lives of others. Not all families choose to do that, which is sad. But many do and find great comfort in it.

It is precisely because this gift is so precious that those involved in the organ donation process want it to go to someone who will take care of it and cherish it for the gift it is.

For that reason, getting on the list takes a series of steps over several months. At Jim's Liver Center, they combine several steps into an all-day bootcamp of sorts where you meet with the variety of people involved in the decision-making process.

Here's what it involves:

Typing and Measurements

Patients receive a liver biopsy. This confirms the initial diagnosis and identifies other factors, which may influence match making. The better the typing done at the beginning of this process, the better the success factors for long-term viability.

One factor is a patient's size. The organ needs to fit today and have room for expansion. Healthy livers regenerate and grow. Sometimes size dictates whether a donated adult liver could be suitable for a waiting child or adolescent transplant patient.

There is also the matter of plumbing. Bigger people usually have bigger connectors (i.e. the arteries and veins which lead to and from the liver). Also, sometimes people have anatomical anomalies — reversed plumbing, if you will. It was as if God was grabbing a bit of lunch when they were made. Or maybe he was daydreaming about refinements to the platypus? These circumstances are not uncommon, and surgeons can adjust for these circumstances during transplant surgery.

Patient Counseling

Jim was told repeatedly that this was a lifelong commitment. This was not a one-and-done thing. He'd need to be ready, willing and able to make lifestyle choices throughout the entirety of his life.

Now Jim is deliberate. He takes planning and commitedness to the next level. Jim was the guy who reminded you that in six-weeks' time, your driver's registration was up for renewal, and your car needed an oil change. He was the guy who bought three months of toilet paper, you know, just in case. (Yes, if you ever need a long, luxurious bathroom trip during the apocalypse or next pandemic, do come to my house.) Jim made sure there were always scissors within reach, and he *never* ran out of tape.

Still, they had no way of knowing this about him, so they asked him question after question:

"If called for transplant, would you stop what you were doing and show up to the hospital?"

Um, yes. I thought, *I think he could put down his phone for that.* It begged the question, do people really ever answer the phone, like, "Sorry, I'm doing an epic stream session on Netflix and just can't go save my life right now."

What we learned was that some people get the call and don't show up. This astonished me. Dozens of people had made choices, taken actions and put careful thought into the extension of your life. You can't even bother to show up? Then I thought of the people, overwhelmed by depression, who might make that choice. I could not imagine being that low in the depths of misery.

"Will you agree to never drink alcohol again?"

Jim said "Yes" without a moment's pause. I am ashamed to say I would have been more hesitant.

This was the first time the liver center had talked about drinking in those terms. Jim had been off the sauce since his diagnosis. But we'd never really had a firm answer on drinking post-transplant. This was the first hard *"No"* we'd heard. No drinking again. Ever.

No New Year's Eve toasts.

No glass of wine with dinner.

Nope.

The thing is, you never realize how much alcohol is part of your life until it's not.

Jim and I had some pretty happy memories throwing a few back over the years. There was a place in Amsterdam called House of Bols that made a local spirit called *Jenever*. We spent one deliriously happy afternoon touring the place and sampling the delicious flavors – *from a heady vanilla to ripe peach.* We sipped our way around, then tipsy-walked all around Amsterdam like college tourists.

Then there were the many times after being out in the Baghdad sun all day when Jim and his work colleagues would drink deeply discounted Johnny Walker Blue scotch chased with handfuls of sesame almonds. They certainly knew how to class up the war zone. Jim — who didn't even like beer — came to enjoy this ritual because it meant hanging out with fun and interesting people whose drinking prowess equaled their storytelling abilities.

For Jim, booze was very much a product of time and place. He drank a little here and there. It never made a good time for him. It was an added dimension to an already good time. It was for that reason, perhaps, Jim felt comfortable putting his drinking days in the rearview.

Family Counseling

Next it was my turn to answer questions…a lot of questions…about how we were doing as a married couple — like *The Dating Game*, except if you got a question wrong, your loved one would die.

I was sweating this meeting. I am not really what one would call the Mother Theresa type. Yes, I generally tried to do good. At this point in my life, though, I hadn't ever had someone else's life truly in my hands. This was one of those moments where I had to double down in the commitment department. A wedding is a party. A marriage is a commitment.

But some questions were actually pretty damned funny.

"Will you drive your spouse to the hospital?"

"Yes. I would carry him if I had to — although a cab might be easier if I couldn't find the car keys."

"Will you be able to decide for him if he is not in a position to do so?"

"Absolutely. Jim's unconscious and I get to call the shots? Sign me up. I do this sort of thing all the time already, like when he is napping and I order my choice of takeout."

"Will you actively support him through this process by regularly accompanying him to transplant center visits?"

"Oh..."

This is where things got a little dicey. Jim was still well enough to get around. Yes, he was tired and had trouble fitting into his pants (Screw you, ascites!), but he was mobile and could have gotten himself here and back on his own steam. The visits were pretty frequent, however, and we were told they would become increasingly so. I needed to adjust my work schedule significantly.

This was probably the first moment I'd realized this would be less a passing inconvenience and more of a life changer.

Financial Counseling

The next stop was the financial counselor. They reiterated a lot of what we'd already heard. This was a lifetime thing. (Check!) This involves significant and recurring expenses. (Check!) This is for the rest of your life. (Yup, we're totally getting that point.)

She also told us the transplant surgery costs $40,000.

Jim and I had prepared for this. We knew transplant surgery would be expensive, even with our uncommonly good insurance. Living was more important than any trip, or any new car, or house, or retirement fund. What were we going to spend it on, anyway? We're two childless homebodies who could no longer invest in a really awesome wine cellar or go skydiving. Our cats might eventually want a totally badass cat tree or a yurt, but we could save up for that. Whatever. We were in.

I took the checkbook out of my bag and said, "To whom do we make it out?"

The financial counselor gave me a funny look. Not a "ha-ha" funny look. More like "bad smell" kind of funny look.

"Did I just do something wrong?"

"No."

"We figured you would want the money."

"No."

I started panicking. *Does she think I'm bribing her? Fuck. Fuck. Fuck. Fuck. Fuck.* I'd just gotten him kicked off the list before he was even on the list. Fuck. Fuck. Fuck. Fuck. Fuck.

"We're not even sure if he is having the surgery yet. When he is called for transplant, we'll put it through insurance first. And then you'll get a bill."

I breathed an epic sigh of relief. "Okay. So, no money today, then."

"No, no money today. And remember, insurance may cover some of those costs. That's my job to find out. Okay?"

That was that. All the information gathered from these visits goes into Jim's file. A board of chosen doctors reviews this file and decides if Jim can go on the list.

Our final meeting of the day was with a member of the surgical team.

While it was Dr. Attia's and her team's job to keep Jim's health stable, it was the surgical team's job to do the transplant itself.

Now, the surgeons take turns, so you are never entirely sure who will be your guy or gal on the day of the surgery. Plus, meeting with a member of the surgical team was unnecessary unless they intended to list you, so I took their scheduling this meeting as a pretty good sign.

Jim and I had spent the past week preparing a really long list of questions in a spiral-bound notebook:

How long is the surgery?

Can I eat salt again? (From Jim, who had a hankering for some real chips and salsa.)

How long do you think he will be on the list? (From me, so I could navigate family medical leave stuff.)

What does recovery look like?

What will happen if I don't receive an organ?

What is the average MELD score at transplant for this hospital?

Our list had 83 questions.

We prioritized the questions. We assumed the doctor wouldn't have much time to spend with us because he or she was, you know, saving lives and all. This was another quirk of coming to the liver center. You would occasionally get, "The doctor is going to be late today because they're doing a transplant." Some patients would groan at this. I never did, because I quietly hoped one day Jim would be the person delaying everyone else's appointments.

In my mind's eye, I figured we'd be meeting someone who had multiple college degrees and a condescending attitude to match.

Instead, we got Dr. Wilcox.

Oh, he had a stellar set of credentials. I also knew him to be among the best in his field. He also, however, had a dazzling smile and a laugh like Dr. Hibbert from *The Simpsons*. He gave us a thorough rundown of what transplant surgery entailed.

While he was giving us the rundown, he must have seen me white knuckling the notebook, because he finally asked: "So, what do you have there?"

"We prepared a list of questions. We figured you'd be busy, so we wanted to be efficient," Jim answered. I nervously began flipping through pages to find our highlighted questions.

"Well, let's hit 'em all!"

True to his word, he did hit them all — Every. Single. One. Here is what we learned:

The surgery itself lasts eight to nine hours. Following that, they keep the organ recipient highly sedated for eight to twelve hours. The purpose is to give the recipient's body time to adjust to the new organ. During this time, doctor's intubate the recipient. Doctors worn transplant recipients to expect this, because when they wake up, the tube might still be in. Dr. Wilcox warned Jim this could feel unnerving. (Like the entire surgery wasn't?) With the tube in, Jim can not speak. But the team works very quickly to take it out.

The donor has his or her own medical team. At many hospitals, there is a brief ceremony of thanks to the donor for giving the gift of life. With the donor family's permission, some hospitals even film this service. I later found some of these touching videos online, with families and medical staff lined up along the sides of the hospital hallway, sharing a moment of silence, as the patient took a final ride.

They call the transplant recipient to the hospital after they have identified a match. After this call, transplant specialists continue to test the donated organ's suitability. What this means is the recipient must prepare for possible disappointment. An unforeseen issue could happen with the gift. My heart broke when I later heard this happened nine different times for one transplant patient. The tenth time, he almost did not come to the hospital because he was so afraid it would end in disappointment. It would seem tenth time was the charm for him.

This thought—that it wouldn't work out—had never crossed Jim's or my mind before. Everything we ever knew about transplants we'd seen in the movies or on TV. For me, it was mainly soap operas. The patient was always wan, with dark circles under her eyes. She had the transplant surgery and within minutes, she was dewy-eyed, rosy-cheeked, back on her feet, and usually in the arms of the sexy surgeon who'd made it all possible. On TV, the patient wasn't told, "Sorry. Go back home. We'll try another day."

We also learned some hospitals identified both primary and secondary recipients. I was always quietly grateful this wasn't the practice at Jim's hospital. I'd been in enough community theater to know what the understudy really thought about the star, and I'd seen the movie *Showgirls* enough times to advise the primary recipient to avoid really tall staircases.

We also learned a liver could live a long time outside the body—up to 16 hours. I imagined his precious gift in a cooler in the passenger seat of a Kia. I wondered what happened if the driver went to pee. Did the driver bring the organ with him? Did he pull out the baby changer shelf in the stall and rest it on there? Did anyone ever try to see what was inside the cooler?

As part of the surgery, doctors open up patients from sternum to the middle of their abdomen. Then the bottom of the incision trees off in two diagonal cuts — one on each side — which goes from mid-abdomen to below the ribs. The incision looks like an upside-down Y. Many patients think it looks like the Mercedes Benz logo, which gave them the double benefit of looking both high class and badass.

"So, what happens if I don't find a match...how...how does that go?" Now, this was the first time Jim had ever talked about his own mortality. You might think this was strange, because that was the first place my mind went: *How fast? How soon?*

Jim was not a spiritual guy. When I asked him about his religious upbringing during our period of modern courting, he'd said, "Mom dragged me to church. By my hair. It was annoying."

As for mortality, Jim was the fiercely practical sort. *I am here. Then I am not.* I think he quietly believed that if Death came knocking at the front door, he would say, "Get off my lawn."

We'd never had a real talk about death beyond the annual life insurance renewal, despite it now being in the realm of higher-than-average probability. I had only recently graduated from the phase of life when you'd lose your grandparents. Jim had gone through the passing of both of his parents. Sure, a meteor could hit us, but that was years off.

But then...this.

This was the meteor.

Jim asking this doctor about how he could die shamed me. I'd never even bothered to ask how he felt about dying. I think I'd just never considered a time when he wouldn't be next to me, watching TV, and bickering about inconsequential stuff.

It took Dr. Wilcox a longer time than usual to consider his answer. Until now, the conversation had been lively and upbeat. He took a deep breath.

"In my experience, people are not so much afraid of dying as they are of pain and the unknown. I think that's why I am matter-of-fact about these things. Sometimes that's the best and only way to give comfort."

He then shared a story about a patient of his from some time ago who did not qualify for a transplant. He didn't share the details, but I got the sense the patient may have revisited the substances he'd probably struggled so hard to avoid.

When that patient had asked Dr. Wilson the same question, he had faced a choice. He could tell a sanitized version, or he could describe, in great detail, what the patient should expect. He went with the truth. "You will become increasingly tired and maybe confused. You will then fall into a coma and quickly fade."

I envisioned a weary soul lying in a hospital bed, hearing the worst news of his life.

"What happened then?" I asked.

"Everything I said came to pass. But he was not afraid. He knew what to expect, and he was not alone. We were all by his side."

That was when I knew we were lucky. Here, we weren't just going to be another name on another file.

CHAPTER 5: OCTOBER

City Hospital, Waiting Room

On Sunday mornings, Jim would hang out with me while I packed my suitcase for my business trip of the week.

"Where are you going?"

"Someplace unglamorous."

"Can I go, too?"

"You can't. You've got a liver to catch."

We were working under the assumption that, barring any *additional* unexpected health anomaly, they would find Jim eligible for transplant. But the factors which governed *when* that would happen were completely out of our hands.

The Family & Medical Leave Act (FMLA) required you to have worked for your employer for a year. You then had twelve months in which to use twelve weeks of leave. You could take days off here and there or in one sizeable chunk. It required the company to maintain your health benefits during that time. What's important to note, however, is that the leave is unpaid.

What this meant in the wonderful world of transplant caregiving was you were constantly playing a game of, "How sick are you...*really?*"

Jim firmly respects "the system." If you follow the steps presented to you deliberately, you will get the desired result.

I never saw it that way. The qualification process spoke of a meritocracy. They added some people to the list while others were not. Some people got to live, others did not.

"I think you're being paranoid about this." Jim told me repeatedly. "I don't have enough experience with this to know whether to be paranoid, so I choose paranoid."

Family support was a dimension of the process that made me more than a little frantic. Using support systems as deciding factors about who got on the list made complete and total sense. The rational side of me got it. The emotional side of me decided the best path forward was epic overcompensation — constant, stomach-churning anxiety about balancing work and caregiving.

I had recently received *the big promotion* at work. Said promotion reflected hard work, luck and circumstances. The company was doing a lot of acquisitions at the time and was woefully shorthanded. I'm a good thinker with a freakishly strong work ethic, and I also was a pleasant travel companion. With this job, you got stuck in a lot of airports, not to mention hours long drives in the snow, stopped trains and missed meals. There's comfort in having a colleague there to watch your bag while you pee and dig a granola bar out of her purse when you are starving.

My job was demanding, but I loved it. I also loved the fact that the medical insurance was keeping Jim above ground and breathing.

While out of town, Jim and I primarily kept in touch via text.

Jim: Hey!
Me: What's up?
Jim: I don't like these new salt-free chips.
Me: What?
Jim: [Photo of potato chip]
Jim: [Photo of cat sniffing potato chip]
Jim: Cato doesn't like them either.
Me: In a meeting, sweetie. Get back to you later, okay?
Jim: I went to get stabbed today.
Me: ?!?
Jim: Monthly blood test.
Jim: New lady. Poked me a bunch. Arm is now sore.
Jim: [Blurry picture of arm]
Jim: Does this look swollen to you?

Jim: I thought it might look a little pink around the edges.
Jim: Should I put antibacterial on it? I have some in my pocket.
Jim: [Picture of cat next to antibacterial]
Jim: Cato is asking if I should?

Jim would never say, "I'm anxious." Instead, he would talk a lot about nothing at all. A two-cat-picture text stream was my cue to step out of the meeting and call him.

"It was such a pain in the ass," he dove in immediately. "When I got there, the room was packed, PACKED. And the parking was awful. I had to park in that distant lot, you know. This is the test they keep over billing us for, too, right? I asked to speak to someone in finance and they said I had to call their help number. I know they process the bills on site. They just didn't feel like talking to me. Well, whatever."

"Are you okay?"

"Yeah, yeah, just fine. I ate lunch a few minutes ago. I really like that new salsa. Who knew you could get salsa without tomatoes? Where has this been all my life?!?"

"I've gotta go back into the meeting. Is there anything else you need right now?"

"I'm good. When are you coming home?"

"Tonight, for me. Early tomorrow for you. Redeye."

"Good. I miss you."

"Miss you, too."

When I got back inside the room, a co-worker familiar with our situation pulled me aside. "It can be so difficult to travel when loved ones need us at home. Is everything okay?"

"He got a bad parking spot and ate tomato-free salsa."

"Huh?"

"Translation: He's fine. Just a little anxious today."

"Ah...got it. I have small boys at home. Same thing."

What helped us on the home front at this point was that Jim could still drive. He could get himself to and from the local blood test place and pick up prescriptions. Places like the grocery store and doctor appointments were a stretch for them. For those, he needed a buddy. Big parking lots and long walks were his new nemeses.

Jim's liver doctors were aware of my travel schedule. I think they found it amusing — doctors and nurses rarely get to travel for work. Patients like Jim need them to stay on home turf.

Whenever his doctors would see me in the lobby, they'd ask: "And where have you been, TJ?"

The Tracey Flick in me wanted to respond with: "Right here by his side the entire time!"

Oh, wait...they weren't judging me, they were being thoughtful and asking about my travel. *London* or *L.A.* always got me a thumbs up. *Johnstown, Pennsylvania,* received a less enthusiastic response.

One thing is true about waiting rooms—everyone there would prefer to be somewhere else. The wait times were long. It was a good day if we only caught three hours of the CBS daytime television lineup while waiting to see Dr. Attia and her team. They blessed us with a long conversation with a doctor when we needed one. Perhaps each day was someone else's day for that gift.

Appointments usually resulted in five or six hours of time lost in the middle of my traditional work day. At first I tried to bring my laptop to these appointments. However, power outlets were few and broadband Internet was unreliable. Also, whenever I unpacked the laptop, many patients would give me the side eye. "Well, don't you think you're so fancy?"

Instead, I made do with sending emails on my phone.

Our House, Dining Room

Jim and I have a sideboard in the dining room, which we use as a bar. The bar has the good/bad distinction of being the first thing you see as you walk in the front door. It is also at the literal center of the home. You can't go anywhere in the house without walking past it.

Jim was off the sauce permanently, and I knew with his steely will, he wouldn't touch a drop. But, wasn't putting a big ole bar in the eyeline of a liver patient like putting a delicious slice of chocolate cake in front of a starving man?

Immediately after Jim's original diagnosis, I boxed up all the liquor and wine in the house and stored it in an office closet. But the bar now looked a little naked. So, I repurposed it.

I ordered two cases of syrup and all the trimmings to go with them. Jim would now be an Italian soda mixologist!

When everything arrived, I shooed Jim into another room and got to work setting up. I got him variations for both club soda and coffee. I unpacked those big pumps they use at your local coffee bar, an old-fashioned straw holder filled with the very finest bendy straws, and fancy shelves that made the bottles look downright decorative. Besides the usual suspects — vanilla, hazelnut, and fruity flavors — I thought a bit outside the flavor box and stocked up on Belgian Cookie, Creme de Cassis, and Mojito.

With my setup finally complete, I unveiled the new bar with all the flourish of a spokes model at a car show.

"What's this?" Jim smiled.

"Your very own bar. Everything on here you can drink."

"Are you serious? Is it good?"

"Well, we'll just have to see, right?"

We got to work experimenting.

Over Italian bubbly for Jim and some Italian vino for me, we got to talking about how this all happened. Jim's diagnosis was Nonalcoholic Steatohepatitis (NASH). We knew that was what had done his liver in, but we didn't really understand *how*.

NASH is caused by three things: obesity (you carry some extra pounds), dyslipidemia (your blood is like butter), and glucose intolerance (your body wants to be candy when it grows up). For those reasons, it's easy to assign blame for NASH. *Perhaps if the patient had put down those deep-fried Oreos he/she wouldn't be in this position?* But if we're all truly honest with ourselves — how often have we reached for a hamburger or bag of candy when a salad would have been better? (Chew on that, Judgy McHighhorse!) I loved wine and believed mozzarella sticks were a food group. Why wasn't I the one who needed a brand-new organ?

It's a not-yet-fully understood combination of heredity, biology and life choices which make some people get NASH and others...not.

"My mom loved cookies," Jim said.

"I know. Her one big vice."

"And she fed me all this terrible-for-you stuff when I was a kid."

"It was the 70s," I tried to reassure him. "We were all weaned on Pepsi."

Halloween, Our House, Living Room

My parents told me my first word was *cookie*. This was followed shortly thereafter by "*costoon*" — my attempt at saying *costume*. This combination was a pretty clear indicator of what my favorite holiday would be.

In an unexpected scheduling boon this year, I got to be at home for Halloween. The day before, I'd gone straight from the airport to the local drugstore to stock up on sweets for trick-or-treaters. Jim examined my haul.

"Really, all that candy?"

"It's Halloween," I said, exasperated.

"That is some NASH waiting to happen."

"What are my other alternatives?"

"I don't know. Toothbrushes?"

"That's what jerks or dentists give out."

He couldn't deny that.

We spent the night on the couch in the living room watching scary movies and enjoying a round of "fauxjitos" (seltzer + mojito-flavored syrup + lime = Yum). Whenever I heard the doorbell ring, I'd throw off the comforter, bolt out of my seat, adjust my wig and witch hat and throw candy by the fist-full into each kid's pillowcase or pumpkin bucket.

"Ever considered apples?" Jim asked.

"Like a toothbrush alternative?"

"Yeah."

"Nope. There was a razor blade thing when I was a kid."

"People gave out razor blades?"

"No, like *in* the apples. By bad people. You never heard of that?"

"Ever considered bottled water?"

"Bottled water for what?"

"To give out."

"That's a good idea, actually. Goes great with candy! I can put some on ice on the porch for kids and parents. We can do that next year."

Then we looked at each other for a moment.

Suddenly, *next year* seemed like a really bold statement.

As we slipped into silence, our hands reached under our blanket to find each other.

CHAPTER 6: NOVEMBER

My Parents' House

Thanksgiving, the holiday centered almost entirely around food, was coming up and I just wasn't feeling it. I wasn't in Grinch territory, but I was in the vicinity. After that strange moment on Halloween I had slid down the slippery slope of thinking of things in terms of the "last" — the last Halloween, the last Thanksgiving, the last Christmas.

I spent all day every day thinking about *The List*. Even when I focused on work or a good tv show, it was always there, lurking. Jim had started the process in July. We'd been told it would take about six months to confirm his eligibility, so it wasn't like we were behind schedule, but we were only into month five and Jim's symptoms were growing increasingly pronounced.

I was a theater kid, however, and what that taught me was that in times of uncertainty, the best move was to smile brighter and shake those jazz hands with even greater enthusiasm. So, instead of curling up in a ball like I wanted to, I took to Thanksgiving with the gusto of a party-planning pilgrim.

Jazz Hands

Thanksgiving this year would be at my parents' house. But to help spread out the work, the meal would be potluck, with everyone contributing a dish or two.

This was the first time many members of the family would see Jim after his diagnosis. They had heard snippets here and there about his situation, but weren't totally in the loop.

"So, what can Jim eat?" My mom asked over the phone in the weeks leading up to the big day.

"Well, it's complicated."

"Can he have Turkey and pie? We'll have lots of turkey and lots of pie."

"Do you have a few minutes?"

I spent the next 20 minutes explaining all the nuances of Jim's diet. It occurred to me that this was the first time I'd ever explained them out loud to another person. I talked about the amount of salt he could have, the average salt milligram amounts in popular foods, special-ordering food on the Internet, making your own condiments, and other helpful advice such as "Canned soup is the Devil's own elixir!"

"So... um, there you have it."

"That's a lot to take in, Toots," my mom said, using my childhood nickname. "So, I guess Cheez-Its are out, huh?"

We then spent another 15 minutes strategizing.

"They make a low-salt Stove Top stuffing, right?"

"Do you want to murder him!?!"

That may have been harsh, but what's important to understand about Jim's restrictions is that things as simple as a grilled cheese sandwich would eat up all of his salt count. The rest of the day would then be all applesauce, carrots, and ice pops.

There's this pendulum in life that has on one side *accommodating* and on the other side *burdening*. In situations like this, you need to figure how far you want it to swing in which direction. My mom and I agreed that asking my cousin to reinvent a green bean casserole without soup or crunchy, yummy onions would break that pendulum right off its hinges.

"A little tablespoon of everything" strategy couldn't work, either. It wouldn't be filling enough for him. Instead, I broke a traditional Thanksgiving dinner into its most basic components:

- Turkey
- Mashed Potatoes
- Gravy
- Stuffing

We would make sure Jim had a nice, normal serving of those, with just enough wiggle room left in his salt count to allow for a sampling of desserts.

My cousin Dee was in charge of the turkey, so I needed to ask her to make some accommodations. Her plan was to do an unbrined bird slathered in salt-free butter. She would salt only the top of the skin — enabling us to cut a few pieces from the middle of the bird for Jim to enjoy.

She was also planning to make a batch of sausage studded, beyond yummy stuffing — the kind people (such as me) wait all year for. In addition, my mom was making her mashed potatoes, which were the stuff of legend — potatoes and milk blended with creamy, creamy butter and salty, salty salt. The consistency was so smooth and fluffy we could pipe them on top of a cake. I couldn't bear the idea of cancelling those meals. We couldn't mess with success. Instead, we would rescue some boiled potatoes and go from there.

The day before Thanksgiving, I turned my attention to making Jim's custom order of stuffing and gravy, or what I was calling Juffing and Jravy.

I started with Juffing. It began by baking low-salt bread in the bread maker. When the bread had cooled, I crumbled it up into small cubes and sauteed it in a pan where I'd already had some finely cut celery and onions cooking. I started adding layers of homemade, no-salt stock I'd made and frozen a few weeks prior. I then added heavy sprinkles of virtually every Mrs. Dash product and a no-salt Garlic seasoning I'd bought in bulk at the warehouse store. For even more flavor and fanciness, I added dried cranberries and unsalted nuts.

As for the Jravy, I cooked down my own homemade stock until it became a bit more concentrated, and then added some white flour to thicken it.

The resulting work, well... let's just say it tasted like love.

The next day, the trip down to south Jersey was short — only about an hour — but it still knocked Jim out. We arrived and immediately settled him in a seat by the fireplace where he spent a good bit of time dozing.

His appearance surprised family who had not seen him for a while.

When we think of the dying, we picture someone wasting away — someone who is skeletal in appearance. Jim looked sallow, but also...just kind of big. It was difficult to understand how this was the man who only ate about one meal a day because that was all his stomach could fit.

When the food came out, Jim joined us at the table. He appreciated the effort everyone had gone to on his behalf. He gave me a big kiss on the cheek, and I made him a big plate. He ate only about a quarter of it.

I could sense the family wanted to ask questions. I think the tendency when you're dealing with a sick person is to smooth it over. "Oh, everything is going so welllllll!" But it was clear to all in attendance that things weren't going, well, well.

After eating, Jim expressed his thanks and asked if we might excuse him. He whispered in my ear he was hoping he might lie down. I helped him up the stairs so he could get a bit of quiet. When I descended the stairs a few minutes later, all eyes were on me. I prepared for the familial interrogation.

Jazz hands

Part of me wanted to come clean — about the illness, about the stress, about my near-constant state of worry, guilt and anxiety. But I was just sick of talking about people being sick.

A few years ago, I'd sat next to a very nice elderly lady at a friend's Passover Seder. My dining companion seemed a little shy at first, but by the time we sliced into our brisket, we were talking like old friends. We discussed interests, opinions, what was good on television, and the last splendid books we read. As we were leaving for the night, she'd given me a big hug.

"That was the best conversation I've had in a really long time."

"Me too! You were lovely company."

"My husband has Alzheimer's..."

"I'm sorry to hear —"

She cut me off with a brisk wave of her hand. "I really don't get out much, and every time I do, the only thing anyone asks about is him. I love him so much. But it's nice to not talk about him sometimes...just once in a while, you know?"

I wished *this* moment could be like *that* moment. Maybe for a few minutes I could forget about our situation and just kind of *be* for a while.

I opened my mouth to speak and felt my eyes water. I looked over at my mother.

She knew just what to do.

"Scratch tickets!" She announced and started handing them out. "I got everyone scratch tickets! Let's see if someone wins big tonight."

My cousin yanked out the seat next to her and pulled me down into it. My other cousin refilled my wineglass to the brim. My dad cut me a slice of apple pie the size of a shoebox.

I tucked into my pie, drank my bubbles, and scratched my ticket. The sounds of family hummed like music.

Facebook Group
Jim's Liver Party
December 8

TJ: "Jim is officially on The List*!!! This means that, once they find a liver of a suitable match and size and a blood type match, he gets* The Call.

The invariable question is...so how long does he have to wait?

The short answer is...it depends.

What does this mean for Jim?

A good bit of waiting. Frequent blood tests are necessary. This is one of the major rules for staying on The List. *He is also under the care of an outstanding and compassionate team of physicians, nurses and transplant coordinators.*

Considering the situation, his mood is good. He always appreciates calls, instant messages, and texts.

What does this mean for us?

Regrettably, our biggest (current) challenge is my travel schedule. I travel all the time for work.

We're managing okay for now. I devote weekends to powering through a week's worth of household tasks. And, my parents have been a godsend. But depending upon how things shake out in the next few weeks, I'm considering bringing in reinforcements to give Jim a hand when I'm on the road (i.e. a good-natured college student who loves talking about politics and cleaning out cat boxes).

How can you help?

If you feel like lending a hand, here are some nice things to do:

1. *Make Jim laugh.*
2. *Offer to be on the phone tree. I may be out of town when we get The Call. I'll need help to get Jim to the hospital and stay with him until I get home.*
3. *Have a glass of wine with me. Jim is off the sauce, but I am very fond of its medicinal powers. It has the added benefit of being cheaper than therapy.*
4. *Be forgiving about our less-than-swell correspondence. Jim falls asleep while eating a sandwich. I'm shoehorning in long-overdue personal emails while waiting in the United lounge at 4:30 a.m. Regrettably, our social skills have taken a major nosedive.*
5. *Sign up to be an organ donor. No, I don't want them now. I would rather *you* keep them. However, when you eventually expire (comfortably, at a ripe old age), you may also be saving someone else's life in the process.*

Well, that's all, folks.

A victory, to be sure.

Now, on to our next battle!"

CHAPTER 7: DECEMBER

Our House

Jim was officially on *The List*. Hope was no longer a tiny, flickering flame. It was a bonfire.

I finally had a license to shift into full-blown preparation mode. Jim and I have one of those really expensive, foamy beds which make you feel as if you're falling asleep cradled by 1,000 angels. My original plan was to turn the main bedroom into "Jim's Recovery Suite." This would give him both quiet and comfort. It had the added benefit of being self-contained. I would clear this room of clutter and bleach it from top to bottom. Then, when Jim eventually came home from transplant, I could essentially wall him off, as this room had both a bathroom and a shower.

This became a no-go when Jim revealed he had trouble getting in and out of our fluffy angel bed. He said it felt too much, as if the bed was sucking him in. He preferred the stiff spring mattress from his first apartment—now in the guestroom. Unfortunately, the bed from our room didn't fit in the guestroom, so it wasn't as simple as swapping the beds. Plan B—I would clean out the guestroom for Jim.

I wasn't a fan of Plan B. The guest room had become the place where we collected "extras," like a less-dusty attic. Even though we had been married for a decade by this point, my mom often treated us like Dickensian waifs, pretending to buy stuff for herself, only to re-gift it to us. "Oops! I just bought myself a second brand-new vacuum by mistake. Would you like this other brand-new one?" On the plus side, as I cleaned, I also discovered there were extra comforters, curtains and two mattress pillow toppers. I was blessing my saintly mother.

It took an entire weekend, but when finished, the room dazzled. I designed the room with great care. Among the highlights: Claw-style grabbers so Jim could pick up anything he'd dropped on the floor, a huge, easy-to-reach nightstand with easy access to power up his devices, a stash of water and salt-free snacks, a space heater because he was always cold, and a sound machine so he could drift off to slumber to the sounds of the beach. I also added a bookcase stocked with with medical equipment, and a selection of easily washable sheets, blankets, and towels.

The finishing touch was a digital photo frame which featured pictures of family, friends and Jim doing things he loved—a little love and motivation all wrapped into one.

When I brought Jim in to see the new room, he smiled. "I love it, honey. Thank you." My heart soared.

He then took a three-hour nap in the just-made bed.

The next challenge was the cats. The cats have a rotation schedule, so one of them is sleeping in our bed 24/7, alternating shifts.

"I'd like to go adopt a cat today," is a sentence uttered by no one ever. People don't decide to get a cat. Rather, a cat just shows up and they rise to the challenge.

Cato (Cat 1) entered our lives when two coworkers walked into the lunchroom holding what appeared to be a loud, wet, tuxedo-wearing squirrel. The squirrel was soon revealed to be a motherless, miniature black-and-white feline of indeterminate sex, found in a parking lot storm drain.

Ever practical, I volunteered to run to the nearby pet store to get some things. I had no idea what those things were, but the in-store staff quickly spotted the wild-eyed woman confusedly wandering the aisles and muttering something about cat food and seized on the economic opportunity. Fifteen minutes later and $200 lighter, I returned to the office to find six grown adults unsuccessfully trying to soothe the now-more-slightly dry bundle of fur.

We took turns trying to feed the wee one. When that progressed with little success, I took the unnamed kitten to a veterinarian I found on the internet.

The doctor declared him a three-week old feline in surprisingly robust health, given his rough start. After I was another $150 lighter, the doctor asked, "You think you are going to keep him?"

I responded with a hopeful yet noncommittal, "Maybe."

That evening, I walked into the house and mutely handed Jim an opened top cardboard box, the contents of which was a scrappy-looking towel and an even more scrappy-looking kitten. Jim then said the most impressively confident sentence I have ever heard a human being utter, "We'll make this work."

We eventually named the kitten Cato after Cato the Younger, a Roman senator. We thought his ever-present tuxedo and frequent use of claws and teeth demanded a name with gravitas. Given his tendency towards sloth and love of a good bowl of anything, names like Fred Astaire were wholly unsuitable.

We thought of YouTube like a third parent. Jim would dutifully brush Cato with a toothbrush, while I took a washcloth and stimulated him to poop. Because YouTube said we should. If YouTube suggested we smear the cat in peanut butter while juggling him under a full moon, we would have done that too. Because if someone with the PurrfectlyPawsome took the time to make a YouTube video of something beneficial for a cat, we would take their and word for it.

Despite our tender, YouTube-inspired care, what we learned over those first few weeks was this: Cato was kind of an asshole.

Yes, he would power snuggle with you in an Olympic medal-worthy way, but he would also play really, really rough. We did the whole "hands and fingers are for feeding and toys are for biting" thing. He loved nothing better than digging his claws into my forearm like a deranged koala and settling in for a nice hang-and-bite. I spent a lot of my time prying Cato off my limbs and slathering myself in antibacterial cream.

What YouTube told us to do was get him a friend. Because cats, the Internet said, learn manners from other cats. Jim went on the hunt for a cat sibling. One day, when he was picking up food for Sir Bites-a-Lot, Jim spotted an adoption event.

One cat caught his eye — a little black one with big, soulful, golden eyes. When Jim reached over for a pet, the cat rubbed his head against the bars in greeting.

"Wow! This cat is really friendly."

"He is, isn't he? Want to hold him?" They sat Jim in a chair and plopped the kitten in his lap. "Such a shame he has three legs. I worry he is going to have a hard time finding a family." Hook, line and sinker.

Jim came home and excitedly told me of his find. "This cat is just something special. It's hard to explain. You just have to meet him."

"Do you think he'll be okay with Cato? Will Cato, you know, rough him up?"

"Maybe they'll be really sweet together?" Jim said, ever the optimist.

So, it was with both hope and trepidation that we made the trip to Petco to pick up Captain Jack. Captain Jack, too, was a foundling. An animal-loving truck driver spotting Jack and his brother at a truck depot. After searching for the kittens' mom without success, the driver called in a rescue organization to assist. The wee brothers still had umbilical cords attached, and Jack's back right leg was in terrible shape. Amputation became a necessity. Now, after several months of care, Jack was finally ready to find a family. Jim had been the very first person to express interest.

We asked the volunteers for tips on how to best integrate our kittens. "Just throw them together and see what happens" seemed to be the consensus.

We came home and went straight into the den, Cato's favorite hangout spot. We took Jack out of the box and plopped him on my lap. Jack burrowed in and made himself at home.

Cato came over and put one foot on my lap before discovering Jack now occupied it.

Cato was normally a quiet cat, but what came out of him was a sustained hiss so powerful we started looking around for Voldemort.

Oh crap, oh crap, oh crap.

Mid Cato's hiss, Jack lazily raised his head from my lap, turned his soulful eyes to his new brother, and paw punched Cato right in the face. No claws. No biting. He just smacked Cato down like a well-trained boxer. Jack then opened his mouth in a jaw-cracking yawn, burrowed deeper into my lap, and started snoring.

Cato, shocked but gracefully accepting defeat, padded over to Jim's lap and settled in for a nice long lap.

We had our matching pair.

Unfortunately, when transplant time arrived, they would need to live away from Jim for few weeks.

I felt bad, so I set them up with a basement bachelor pad. I collected extra rugs, cat beds, bowls and cat boxes.

The basement stairs were steep, and even with help, Jim could not get up and down them. Eager to show off my handiwork, I made an MTV "Cribs" style video to show him all the features — private bathroom, multiple bedrooms, scratching pole, catnip aromatherapy station. All that was missing was a refrigerator of Crunk juice.

The last item on our transplant prep list was deciding on a name for the soon to be an occupant of Jim's body — his future liver. Names had power, and we needed a powerful name. "*Jim's Hoped-For New Liver*" wasn't cutting it.

"What about Oliver?" I asked.

"Like 'Oooohhhhh liver!'"

"Like from The Brady Bunch too, right?"

"The one that moved in."

"Yeah, to save the show. You know, 'Cousin Oliver.'"

"Wasn't the show canceled after that?"

"Yeah, but not, like, immediately."

"Do you think it is bad luck to name a new organ after a character on a cancelled TV show?"

"I wouldn't worry. I think you hit your bad luck quota for this decade already."

The days leading up to Christmas were much calmer than Thanksgiving. Jim wasn't up to traveling and I wasn't up to hosting. The family sent gifts for us, so on Christmas morning I handed them to him to open by the light of our miniature tree.

Unable to shop, Jim gifted me with a set of his mother's pearls that I wore the rest of the day, dressing up my sweatpants.

Dinner was simple, a bit of meat, veggies and potato, but I went all out on the dessert—making a Pear Tarte Tatin from scratch—because it was Jim's favorite.

After dinner, we sat in front of our electric fireplace, Jim under a blanket and with cats in our laps.

"This is pretty nice, isn't it?"

"Yes, it is. It is."

CHAPTER 8: JANUARY 1-17

Clothing Store Near Our House

Tarte Tatin aside, Jim usually stuck to a diet of baked chicken breasts and carrots.

Nevertheless, his weight kept going up and up. It had become a genuine struggle to find clothes that fit him.

Sweatpants were the easiest — easy up, easy down. Who wanted to mess with buttons and zippers when they felt like crap on toast? Socks were challenging. His feet were always cold, but the elastic pinched and felt itchy. Shirts were the biggest problem. The best way to describe it was Jim's head, neck, and arms were regular-sized. His toes to mid-thighs were regular-sized. But the middle of him was about 4X larger than the rest of him.

We finally found a clothing store near us which catered to men of larger stature. I brought Jim there so we could pick out some stuff. Jim was very deliberate about his clothing choices. The thought of me going there and buying him stuff without him trying it on was so ludicrous he couldn't imagine it.

I was a bit of a clothing store novice. I bought all my stuff from the same place — one where I'd stand in a room and a lady more stylish than me would hand me things to try on. I'd take the stuff that fit to the register, pay, and leave. Did I mention my favorite store only sold clothes in two primary colors? I barely ever shopped for myself, and I've never shopped for clothes for Jim. So, despite our marital longevity, this was a fresh experience for us.

When we walked in the door hand-in-hand, Jim huffing and puffing, me looking like a fish on a tricycle, the two-member staff probably guessed we weren't there for holiday returns.

I briefly explained the situation. Transplant. Clothes. Comfort. A dangerous risk of going naked.

The kindly lady suggested Jim have a seat, and we'd bring stuff over to him for examination. Because even though there might be only one shirt in the world that fit him, Jim would still complain about button placement.

At that point, I would have classified Jim's dressing style as *Necessity Chic*. He'd wear the pair of sweatpants with the fewest holes, several layers of shirts with a fleece (unzipped, thanks to ascites belly) and a hat. Jim wore a hat both indoors and outdoors because he was always cold. Today he was wearing a porkpie hat — his *"We're going to the doctor today!"* hat.

The team at the store observed Jim from head to toe. I think they interpreted the hat as a nod to Latin style and flair, so they started bringing him the equivalent of church clothes and *sassy sensual night on the town* wear. While Jim politely fended off their ministrations ("No, I don't salsa dance, but thank you," Jim said while turning down a palm tree-accented, short-sleeved dress shirt), I ran around the store grabbing whatever looked comfortable and easy to get on and off.

Shirts. Pants. Sweaters.

When the team saw what I was grabbing, they followed suit and came up with some nice picks. It was like that scene in *Pretty Woman* — only with a 40-something man and the attentive staff bearing armloads of cotton shirts.

The woman on the team, whom I learned was the store manager, also gently nudged me toward undergarments and accessories. "Guys keep buying the same-sized underwear and wonder why it feels uncomfortable. From what you're saying, he has probably gone up a size or two."

She also pointed out some socks which might feel better on his growing legs.

She then asked, "Does he have a bathrobe? Come feel these."

She led me to a rack of 4X bathrobes. I touched one. It had that magical quality my mom calls *"the gooshy."* It's when an item of clothing or bedding feels so touchable and soft, it must have been handcrafted by angels.

I grabbed a robe for Jim to try on.

By this point, the man on the team had directed Jim to the changing room. Jim was a frugal man. He bought things sparingly because he didn't like clutter. He'd wear one shirt until it had holes in it, but the truth of the matter was, I wasn't sure how often I could get back to this store. I needed to stock up.

"Whatever he likes, I'd like to get two of everything, please. But, could you ring it up...um, quietly?"

This was clearly not the first time this store manager had been to this rodeo. Jim emerged from the dressing room right around the time they'd started ringing up the order. My plan was to shoo him out to the car, finish the checkout, and deposit the bags in the trunk. Then I would take the receipt and throw it in the fires of Mount Doom, never to be seen by Jim again.

"I've got this covered. Why don't you head out to the car?"

"I'm all good. We can head out together."

Dammit.

In the time Jim was in the fitting room, the heap had gotten pretty big, to include belts, an extra bathrobe, lots of undies, socks, a half a dozen shirts and pants, a jacket and a polar fleece.

I watched her ringing things up, and the ticker started getting up there, like *really* up there. We didn't have the luxury of time to go to a bunch of different stores. Shopping here today met a need, and I was happy to spend our dough at a store where the staff was so kind and helpful.

Then Jim saw the total. "But I don't need that many clothes."

"Yes, you do. We can't have you going around all naked." I was serious about this. We'd almost had to have him wear a shirt as a sarong to a blood draw the other day.

"Oh...but I haven't added the coupons in yet." The manager suddenly chimed in.

"Coupons?"

"You remember. The ones you gave me a few minutes ago."

Seriously. I hadn't given her any coupons. We had never been to this store before.

"And we have our post-Christmas sale going on, too. Let me ring in those discounts."

Now, my husband loves value. Like, wants to hug it. Coupons are better than Christmas to him. As the price kept dropping, my husband started patting me on the back. "Good couponing, honey!"

The end of the transaction was about 50% less than when it started. Jim now had the first spring in his step I'd seen in a while. I handed him some lighter bags and asked him to go heat up the car while I grabbed the rest.

"I don't know what you did, but I can make up the difference now."

The manager instead touched me on the shoulder and said, "Honey, we all have to look out for each other. Now, you go enjoy those new clothes with your man. I hope things work out for you guys."

When I got in the car, I blamed my misty eyes on the cold.

Facebook Group
Jim's Liver Party
Tuesday, January 9

TJ: "Bit of an update: At Jim's monthly doc visit this morning, doc hospitalized him to improve his kidney function. Being admitted to the hospital now and will know more tonight and tomorrow. Jim is in good spirits and eager for a nap."

City Hospital, Liver Center, Examination Room

There was now a rhythm to our liver center visits. Jim and I would arrive. He would sit. I would get him checked in. When they called his name, he would walk to the scale and get weighed. His ascites were very pronounced, so he had difficulty maintaining his balance. I would help him take off his multiple layers of outerwear, and a member of the medical staff would help him on the scale.

The nurse looked at his weight and compared it to his chart. "It's a little higher than last time." This was where one would customarily insert a joke about too many Christmas leftovers, but there were none of those this year. The only thing Jim had felt like eating this week was frozen fruit pops and salt-free salsa. He was an accidental vegan.

After the weight, there was always a wait (insert rim shot here) and the doctor would come in to review Jim's blood test results.

It was a different doctor this week, one we had never seen before. She introduced herself, asked how Jim was feeling, and then started flipping through the printout of the blood test results.

"Hmmmm..."

One never likes to hear that sound coming from a doctor.

Since this was her first time seeing Jim, we figured (read: hoped) it might be an introduction *"hmmm"* versus an alarmist *"hmmm."*

"Is there a problem?"

"Have you ever had problems with your kidneys?"

What the what now?

"I just don't like what I'm seeing here. Give me a minute. I'll be right back."

Kidneys are a pair of organs in the back of the abdomen. Each is about the size of a fist. Kidneys remove waste and control fluid balance in the body. They also regulate the balance of electrolytes. Kidneys do this by filtering blood. The liver's principal job is to filter blood from the digestive tract before it circulates through the rest of the body. As Jim's liver decompensated, his kidneys began picking up more of the load. They had stepped up to become the 24-hour cleaning crew.

"Honey, are you feeling okay? Peeing okay?"

"I feel good. And you know I never pee." Translation: I feel as crappy as yesterday, and I still hold my water like a desert camel.

The doctor reentered the room with a stack of papers in her hand. She looked as if she was on a mission. "We're going to need to admit you."

"...to the hospital?" Jim asked, alarmed.

"...like now?" I added dumbly.

"His Creatinine is dangerously high. We feel this is the best course of action."

When a transplant center doctor uses the word *dangerous*, you know shit is getting real.

"I'm calling this in right now. They're going to get a wheelchair for you. Why don't you grab a seat in the lobby until they get here?"

She directed us out and started coordinating with the staff.

"So, this is a little unexpected," I said in the unsettling quiet the doctor left behind.

"I guess this means I'm really sick, huh?"

"Seriously, how do you feel? Different from yesterday?"

"Still crappy, and no."

The wheelchair and driver arrived.

"You know, I can walk there. I mean, I walked in here."

"It's that wheelchair insurance thing. Just roll with it." I said with a hollow laugh.

"Honey, we don't have any of my stuff." By that, Jim meant his tablet and power charger.

"I have to figure this is a give you IV meds and send you home kind of thing, right?" I said hopefully.

They wheeled him out of the liver center with me by his side. Admissions for the hospital was in the lobby which, interestingly enough, we had never seen. The liver center was in the hospital complex, but not in the main hospital building. The utility of the wheelchair quickly became apparent as I ventured forth on a brisk mile-long walk. I panted by the time we reached the destination.

There are two ways to check in to the hospital — Admissions and the Emergency Room. Admissions means, "Hello! You're expecting me." Emergency means, "Holy shit! Um...hi."

Now, just because the hospital said they want you to do something right away doesn't actually mean they can accommodate you *right away*. After being wheeled down to admissions, we were told the wait could be awhile. I later learn that *"awhile"* in hospital terms means anywhere from two to six hours.

The lobby was a bit of a contrast to the rest of the hospital—a cavernous, warm, light-filled place. It was so warm Jim actually took off one of his coats.

It was now getting to be around 2 p.m. and we hadn't eaten since about 7 a.m. that morning. I wished hospitals issued buzzers, much like TGIFriday's. Even though there are not many places to go within the confines of a hospital, it would be nice to have the freedom to get a coffee in the cafeteria while you wait "awhile."

At 4 p.m., they admitted Jim.

City Hospital, Liver Ward

This was Jim's first hospital admission since his diagnosis, and his first medical episode since getting on The List.

During his first hospital visit, Jim had been an oddity. For this visit, patients surrounded him whose condition matched his own. These doctors and nurses were fluent in liver. There was something powerful in being understood without having to explain yourself.

Jim's weight gain was clearly ascites. You could use shorthand with the doctors and nurses, which felt liberating. Despite the scary situation, we were members of the club. The doctor on duty confirmed that Jim's Creatinine was through the roof. His kidneys—which had been such brave soldiers in this battle — were crapping out.

"So, what does this mean?"

"It means we have to get your kidneys in better shape."

"Is that possible?"

"There are lots of things we can do and we're going to do them."

"What happens if my kidneys fail?"

"Well, we will do everything in our power to avoid that happening." We were used to straight-talking doctors. This positive-but-vague treatment was new and a red flag that some serious stuff was going down.

Compromised kidneys are one thing which can push up a MELD score. In an ideal scenario, what that would mean is that Jim would — fingers crossed — get transplanted right away. Not having to cover for Oliver (aka the new liver), the kidneys could recover.

Severely compromised kidneys could have their own series of unhappy outcomes, including Chronic Kidney Disease or renal failure. The former was a lifelong condition which requires constant care and potentially a subsequent transplant. The other meant death.

We had never really thought about kidneys before. We knew about as much as your average person did. People had two but could survive with one. Hence, a living donation was possible. We knew folks with diabetes were often challenged to keep theirs in good health. Dialysis, the cleansing of one's blood using specialized machines, was something which regularly saved and prolonged lives but was best avoided.

What had helped keep Jim in the "Wow, you're just really unhealthy" versus "OMG, you're totally going to die" emotional range was that his kidneys had been powerful performers.

Well, not anymore.

Enter Team Kidney.

Jim's room was at the end of a long hallway. I stepped outside for a moment, just in time to see a formidable group strutting down the hall. It was fronted by an impossibly good-looking blond doctor and flanked by a team of other doctors. They all walked in this determined way, like a pack on a mission. When they passed under a heating vent, their hair and lab coats caught the air and blew around dramatically. *Back in Black* suddenly started playing in my mind.

Those doctors are going to kick the ever-loving ass of whatever is messing up one of these patients, I thought.

They were coming closer and closer to where I stood at the end of the hall when they made a sharp right into Jim's room.

Oh yeah, I thought. *We have Fucking Got This.*

City Hospital, Jim's Room

The bad news about Jim's kidney gave him a higher MELD score, but the high MELD was an unexpected gift. Patients on the waiting list provided blood samples, and the doctors submitted them to UNOS. The list gets updated once a week. Given the timing of Jim's kidney extravaganza, he got his best/worst (depending upon how you look at it) MELD score in his entire liver career — a 28 — at the start of a new week. That meant he had a better chance of being selected for a transplant this week than ever before.

That is one of the many surreal things about waiting for a transplant—you're elated when your loved one is sick enough to be on the tippy top of the waiting list for transplant but well enough to carry on a normal conversation with you—albeit in a hospital, attached to lifesaving drugs, wearing a felt hat, and under enough blankets to suffocate an ox.

I got pretty good at reading the publicly available UNOS online database, and because Jim had some unique attributes—namely age, blood type and cause of illness, it was pretty easy for me to find "him." I was over the moon at his position. This was the first time a transplant wasn't a distant hope but a real possibility. This could be the Hollywood-style ending. The first visit to the hospital since the diagnosis and just as his kidneys failed — a miracle.

I got drunk on hope. I pictured myself standing by his bedside, holding his hand while the doctors told Jim the miraculous news.

But we weren't quite there yet. It was time for doctors to continue their work while Jim focused on recovery.

Facebook Group
Jim's Liver Party
January 13

TJ: "Jim is hanging tight at MELD 28. (There's some math here about Creatinine down and INR up. But I'll spare you the deets.)"

Last night, Jim puffed up. The good doc says this is a natural response to the kidney therapy. Today they're addressing the problem with IV diuretics. (Lots of peeing.) Tomorrow, doctors will switch Jim to oral diuretics. (A little less peeing?) Provided nothing weird happens — or Jim gets The Call about a brand-new liver — Jim should be home on Wednesday. I'm headed up to see him tomorrow morning. (I can listen to stories about his peeing?) We will continue to keep you posted on Jim's progress.

City Hospital, Jim's Room

Think about a gallon of milk. That's about four pounds. Jim's weight could fluctuate one to three gallons of milk within 72 hours. Think about the burden that puts on your body.

Fat has a gelatinous quality to it. It's heavy and uncomfortable, but it stays put. I certainly have enough of it to be an authority on the matter. Fluid is different. It finds an open space at your lowest center of gravity and moves there. That explained Jim's enormous belly.

Even getting up to go to the bathroom was a time-consuming, exhausting ordeal. Dangle over the side of the bed. (Slosh.) Scoot the IV pole closer. (Slosh.) Plant both feet on the ground. (Slosh.) Slow rise to your feet. (Slosh.) Put one foot in front of the other and repeat until you reach your destination. (Sloshy, sloshy, slosh, slosh.)

Jim was never much for bathroom breaks. He could hold his water for ages. This became a very useful skill in Iraq, which wasn't the land of highway rest stops. But for the first time, he had the bladder of a 50-year-old woman after bearing 10 children.

Doctors gave Jim a diuretic called Lasix. The name might ring a bell because it's what they give racehorses to make them "pee like a racehorse" before a horse race.

Jim took to sending me text reports throughout the day about his prodigious pissing. There's nothing quite like being in the middle of a meeting and having your phone show a picture of a triumphant thumbs up next to a just-flushed toilet.

Facebook Group
Jim's Liver Party
January 14

TJ: "The daily dispatch... They are still working on the fluid problem. (Jim feels like a slightly deflated whoopie cushion. He also has Fred Flintstone feet.) Doctors keep pushing the diuretics while monitoring Jim's kidneys. Hospital discharge date keeps getting pushed out. Tomorrow is possible; Thursday is more likely. Jim is currently bunking in the ward for trauma patients (e.g. car accident victims, unfortunate bullet recipients). Given that, Jim's condition represents a change of pace for the medical staff, so they don't seem to mind keeping him around. Jim *likes the team but doesn't share their opinion regarding his length of stay.*"

City Hospital, Jim's Room

Jim's unexpected extended hospital stay made him a little homesick. So, the plan was for me to head to the hospital after work so we could have a date night — hospital style.

At that point, I was living on grilled chicken sandwiches from the nearest fast food establishment, bolted down in the car on the way to or from somewhere. Because Jim's diet was so restricted, I felt bad eating anything in front of him. For date night, I made an exception. I would bring something with me to his room for my dinner and Jim would save his dessert, so we could dine together.

Jim is a talker and, most of the time, I am a good listener. But, dog tired and barely able to stay awake, let alone have a meaningful discussion about medical treatment and heavier topics, like fleeting mortality.

Jim needed to focus all of his energy on staying alive. This meant he had to find joy and excitement in everything, even mundane things. After a while, mundane things become the rule rather than the exception, because when one is sick, your world becomes quite small.

I think that's why healthy people get frustrated talking to sick or elderly people, because what sparks joy varies. With a healthy, well-rested mind, I can modulate to that. But, with an exhausted mind and body, I have a tendency to get snappish.

While the sick must think small to survive, the well caregiver has to keep the enterprise running. What the sick then miss is all the behind-the-scenes planning the well take on — the daily administration of illness. Today my task was to battle through my tiredness and impatience. It was time to paste on my best pageant smile and ask Jim about his day.

Spoiler alert: It was a urination celebration.

Jim sipped on an elementary-school-style carton of milk and nibbled on a sad-looking brownie. I swigged a Diet Dr. Pepper while wolfing down a hospital-made sandwich of unknown providence.

As Jim shared his adventures in urination, I tried desperately to mask my yawns as "Oh, urine!" excitement faces.

"Honey... you look really tired," Jim finally said.

"No. I'm not at all tired." I protested.

"You're lying."

"No, really. I'm all good. Let's talk," I tried to say through another enormous yawn.

He gave me a pitying stare. "How about we watch some TV?"

My eyes moved over to the TV mounted to the wall. I pictured the grainy reruns of *Charmed* and local news that would be available and wasn't terribly excited.

Jim read my mind and instead positioned his tablet on his dinner tray. I slid my guest chair closer to the head of the bed and pulled up another chair for my feet. His bed made a low whirring sound as he lowered it to my level.

Jim popped open the HBO app and the familiar notes of the *Game of Thrones* theme song started playing.

Jim shared some of his extra blanket, and for the first time in a while, I felt cozy.

A nurse entered to do some tests and looked askance at our seating arrangement.

"We're on a date!" Jim explained happily.

The nurse laughed. "Well, you need mood lighting then, don't you?" She flipped off all the lights in the room. "These tests can wait," she said. "I'll see you in an hour." She winked and shut the door behind her.

"Quick, let's make out!" Jim said conspiratorially.

I smooched his cheek, and we held hands while watching the Mother of Dragons do her thing.

"Man, I really hope I live to next season."

Facebook Group
Jim's Liver Party
January 16

TJ: "Jim got green-lighted for discharge today. I spent the day there getting him sorted. Here's the scoop:

He ended his stay in the Liver Ward. Before he departed, the liver surgical team stopped by to check if his condition was still good for surgery. (It is!)

This also happened:

Chief Liver Surgeon to Primary Liver Doctor: 'You're discharging this guy???'

Primary Liver Doctor: 'See for yourself.'

Jim appears to be the most lucid, cheerful MELD 28 pointer they have ever encountered.

As we were leaving the hospital, the nurses were going, 'See you soon!' Only in transplant land is that not weird. (Okay. It's still kind of weird.)

As I write this, the no-longer-a-patient is resting comfortably. I'm not sure if he was more excited for his own bed or to see the cats.

I'll be working from home tomorrow, as Jim remains unsteady on his feet. A combination of masquerading as a water balloon and blood-pressure lowering drugs have a way of doing that to you. Thank you for your continued support. Stay tuned and pray for a match!"

Our House, Home Office

In the United States, about 20 people die every day while waiting for a life-saving transplant. A match was not found in time. For some people, the wait is especially long. It is not uncommon for a kidney patient to wait five years or more to receive the gift of life.

Waiting for a transplant differs greatly from getting treatment for other medical conditions. With other conditions, there can be a lot of unknowns and question marks. With organ transplantation, you know exactly what is wrong. You know exactly what you need to fix it, but you can't get what you need to fix it. It's a matter of supply and demand.

Imagine is someone says to you, "We can cure your cancer. All you need is this one pill. But we can't decide if you will or won't get it. We'll call you if and when you can have it."

There's no way around it — when you have a loved one on the waiting list, you begin to look at generosity and death differently.

I found it gratifying when people heard of Jim's condition and said, "I'm a registered organ donor." My standard response was, "He would prefer you keep your own organs for now, but thanks so much for your kindness. You're doing something wonderful." Their response was unsolicited, which made it nice.

However, for every person who would say those kind words, there would be another who would — unsolicited — say, "No, I'm not an organ donor. It's just not for me. Can you understand what I'm saying?"

No. No, I can't.

They sought validation. They wanted me to make them feel better about their choice. I was busy helping my husband manage his imminent demise. I didn't have time to debate them on this. Also: Did they really just say that to someone whose family member is on the organ transplant waiting list?

My response? "Well, it's your choice. Gotta go! I'm off to the hospital again. Because, you know, dying relative and all. Bye!"

Hope made me judgmental of others and greedy for my loved one's life. I felt myself becoming bitter and knew it was time to broaden my support system.

I found some message boards that were helpful in getting a better understanding of symptom management. For example, I could get a rough estimate of how long someone may be in the hospital if they are a liver patient and their kidneys had issues.

Doctors are very good at dealing with the *now*, especially with transplant patients. Doctors look at each day in isolation, trying to get the best outcome for that 24 hours, and then an even better outcome for the *next* 24 hours, and so on.

Our doctors were not as good at giving us an outlook into what our next week or month might look like. The message boards filled that gap. As a caregiver, knowing what to expect was essential for making plans. For example, if a certain ailment had someone's wife in bed for two weeks, I knew I'd need to adjust my work schedule so I could be home if the same thing happened to Jim. It was imperfect, of course, but it was better than dealing with an informational black hole.

Jim didn't go on the message boards and largely avoided any examination of his condition in any detail. This frustrated me. He had more time on his hands than I did. Why wasn't he looking up this stuff?

I realize now it just takes special energy and focus to distract yourself from dying.

While I was educating myself, Jim was on the wellness track. He'd set out to be a star student in the liver department. No, he wasn't doing extra research, but if his doctors or nurses told him to do something, he would do it and do it well. By excelling at every task in front of him, he could at least have the satisfaction in a job well done. Even if the worst happened, he could say he tried.

CHAPTER 9: JANUARY 18

Our House, Front Yard

Friday and Saturday were pretty tame this week by waiting transplant family standards. Jim hibernated while I did laundry and dealt with everyday stuff. Snow was on that list.

My ever-practical parents had bought Jim and me a snowblower one year as a Christmas present. But snowblowers are temperamental. They may not have gas. They may still have the gas you put in last year and forgot to burn off. The mix might be off. Sometimes the snow is unsuitable to blow.

I'm talking about snow boulders.

One of the great things about living in the suburbs is trucks will come by in the night and make your streets look pristine. The unfortunate consequence is all the stuff that was in the road is now at the bottom of your driveway, effectively making a solid snow barrier that blocks you from actually getting onto the expertly plowed street.

I used to have this dream where Jim got *The Call* during a snowstorm and we had to get to the hospital. I had a few backup plans in my mind. The first line of defense was to actually let Jim drive. He was wildly uncomfortable, but he was a superb driver in hazardous conditions (See: Iraq). I'd be his trusty navigator and he would be the badass patient. If we got pulled over, he would get to say: "I am driving myself to the hospital to get a new liver. Mind speeding this up?"

The back-up was my friend Reagan. Because she was just that kind of crazy. She also knew everyone in town and could make anyone do anything by offering them her home-cooked pork loin.

The doomsday scenario was that I would call the local rescue squad and plead my case. They had:

1. an ambulance
2. kind volunteers who knew how to drive said ambulance
3. a sense of adventure.

I gathered that, between them and the police, we would somehow find our way an hour north.

The more common scenario was we would have a somewhat everyday need (prescription refill, trip to the doctor, blood draw) and I would need to get us there on our own steam. I didn't want to be the girl who cried snow — using up all my favors.

When I was out of town on business trips, the fabulous Jake aided us. He'd use our blower to clean off our driveway and walkways, then do his own house and his parents' before returning the snow blower to us. We covered all gas and related costs. We would have liked to have done more, but Jake wouldn't accept payment.

At one point, he confessed he was nursing a rather serious groin injury. I then pictured him doing his best cowboy walk while shoving the snow guzzler up the driveway. While we were grateful for his help, we preferred he sit at home with a nice, big ice pack on his Johnson.

So, most of the time, snow clearing duty fell to me. We lived in a modest little ranch home. If you close your eyes and picture a suburban house from one of the 1980s Steven Spielberg movies — like where E.T. lived during his earth sojourn — you would get a good picture of our domicile.

In between chores, I would check in on Jim and offer liquids (which he could only drink sparingly) and food (for which he just didn't have a taste) and cats (which he would never turn down).

By this point, I settled Jim in his new guestroom-turned-bachelor-pad across the hall. By "settled," I mean I smothered him under four comforters in a room heated to Aruba-like conditions.

I was working full-time, caring full-time, running back and forth to the hospital, worrying constantly, trying to make our home life not suck by celebrating holidays, cooking reasonable meals for people on special diets and trying to be a phenomenal pet parent. Snow turned out to be the unpredictable variable that could tip a day from difficult-to-manage to impossible-to-manage.

I also had an unspeakable rage for my neighbors. Back when Jim was whole, and I was not a zombie, we used to be the kind of folks who would shovel other people's walkways. If I had the blower out, why not help someone else? We would do a big twirl around the block so everyone would benefit from a clean sidewalk.

Now, when I really needed help, my neighbors had forsaken me. They would do the suburban move of shoveling right up to the property line. They had no obligation to shovel me out. But, at that point in my life, my neighbors going a few feet past the property line would have done tremendous good for my fragile morale.

Late night drives to/from the airport or to/from Jim's medical appointments were the hardest for me to stay awake during. For the first half hour of the drive, I would run on pure adrenaline. It was that last half hour in the cold and dark which was the killer.

I tried listening to podcasts, but there's nothing like listening to people talk about things they enjoy, but you can't do. I loved audiobooks, but they made me sleepy.

Energy drinks were okay in a pinch, but I used them sparingly because they made me alert for hours. Cocaine and heroin were out, too, because, you know, illegal and bad for you and whatnot. Also, it was hard enough getting one liver. I wanted to avoid needing two. I needed a creative solution. That's when the thought came to me — *music*.

To help me stay awake and alert, I would try to remember school choir songs. I was a big fan of choir. I was a serious introvert who also liked to sing. The two rarely go hand-in-hand. Choir gave me the anonymity which the shyness craved, while also letting me unleash my inner Ethel Merman. Plus, don't jazz hands just look so much better when another hundred-and-fifty children were doing them, too? Participation in school music programs also got me out of two days of gym per week.

Trying to remember the lyrics brought me back to life's easier times and also engaged my brain in a way which disallowed sleep. Very useful, that. During this period, I taught myself every single word from a variety of musicals. The soundtrack of *Dr. Horrible's Sing-Along Blog* became one of my first and very best companions.

Our House, Living Room

Hospital visits were exhausting. The rule of thumb is that for everyday you're in the hospital, it takes two-to-three days at home to recover. So, Jim had about a month's worth of exhaustion all stored up.

It was hard for him to stay awake and engaged. When we talked, it was transactional. I would also sometimes read him silly news posts from Facebook, as he didn't feel like watching TV or doing much else. His state of being was as bad as your most dramatic friend describing her case of mono — multiplied by 100.

Everyone's liver is different, and everyone's liver failure is different. Jim's was incredibly uncomfortable and highly debilitating, but mostly pain-free.

Then, on Sunday, Jim was lying on the couch watching football. It was the NFL Playoffs. Jim didn't look as if he was enjoying himself, but it wasn't about the game. He had an odd look on his face, one I hadn't seen before.

"How are you feeling?" I asked.

"Weird. Just weird."

"Can you contextualize that a bit for me?"

"I feel not good."

"You're a liver patient. 'Not good' is, like, every day."

Then Jim didn't so much as smile. We had agreed to go full stupid on this. If there was amusement to be had, we would have it. We would make terminal liver disease fun, dammit!

But this. This guy. This guy right now. He was not my guy.

I helped pull him to a sitting position and dropped to my knees on the floor next to him. "Does it hurt anywhere?"

"My belly."

"Like, 'I'm full' hurt?" I asked, thinking of his bladder and also ruling out the possibility that a big poo would fix all of this.

"Not exactly."

"Hurts like, 'I'm going to hurl,' hurt?"

"No. It's pain. Just pain."

I went for the thermometer. Higher than normal, but not OMG high. Jim's hands gravitating towards his belly and I reached for the phone.

In transplant land, there is always a doctor on call. I hoped we could get some resolution over the phone for this. A doctor saying "This is normal" or "I'll call in a script for this," would ease Jim's mind and help us resolve this quickly.

Unfortunately, while the doctor didn't sound immediately alarmed, she directed us toward the Emergency Room. I asked her which one. Her suggestion was — if he could make the drive — we should go to the City Hospital Emergency Room.

"Oh, jeez. I just wanted to watch some football," Jim said with chagrin, accompanied by a wince.

I quickly gathered the things we would need, endeavoring to be much better prepared this time. I put Jim's tablet, charger, extension cord, electric blanket, and Chapstick in his bright red Manchester United bag, zipped it up and threw it over my shoulder.

Jim felt a great deal of pain moving around. So, the plan was to use comforters to pad the back seat so he could find a position in which felt comfortable and — if he was lucky — try to get some shuteye on the way to City Hospital.

The drive was harrowing. Jim didn't just notice every bump, he *experienced* them. He tried to stay quiet, but the pain became too much and a string of *"Ow"s* escaped. A reflexive apologizer, each Jim "Ow" was followed by me saying, "Sorry!" This chorus and refrain continued throughout the whole hour-long drive.

City Hospital, Emergency Room

Emergency Rooms cater to the desperate — the desperately ill and the desperately poor. This goes double for city-based emergency rooms, which serve the most vulnerable of patients. Emergency Rooms are an odd collection of maladies. The case of sniffles could be one curtain away from a fall off a ladder or an accidental overdose.

Jim didn't fare well in triage because he was absent chest pains or a gaping wound. When they weren't doing transplants, this served as the region's foremost trauma hospital. So, Jim sat amongst the sprains and juicy coughs and waited as patiently as one can while they are dying.

Every minute that went by, Jim clutched his belly tighter, hunching his shoulders. By the end of several hours of waiting, he was practically in the fetal position. The best I could do was try to warm him up in the drafty waiting room.

Finally, he got the privilege of a bed. As Jim curled into a ball, trying to not audibly whimper, I got the distinct impression transplant patients weren't *de rigueur* here in the Emergency Room.

When a resident doctor came in to get his medical history, I gave her the speech I had prepared during the hours of waiting. Transplant patient. Abdominal pain. List of drugs. List of doctors' names at the hospital. Status of food and drink. Dates of most recent hospital stay.

She then asked what I thought was the most important question of all. "James, how much pain are you in? 1 is mild. 10 is the worst pain you have ever been in."

His face contorted from discomfort. "I would say a 9 or 10."

"Well, we'll get you something for that right away."

"Thank you," Jim said between grunts. He looked relieved.

Feeling he was in expert hands for the moment, I headed out in search of the ladies' room. With no signs or a hospital employee in sight, I had to choose my adventure. Out through two double doors, a turn to the right, a turn to the left. Suddenly, I nearly collided with the human form of a brick wall.

Well over 6′4″, this gentleman had the look of someone with whom you wouldn't want to tangle. He dressed casually, but with enough carefully selected gold and diamond accessories that he either sold jewelry or, perhaps, less legal products.

"Oops. Apologies for that. I was just looking for the — "

"Bathroom? Right over there." He pointed to a well-marked door about eight feet away.

"Thank you for your help." I turned and walked toward the door.

"I'll make sure no one bothers you."

This seemed an odd thing to say about a ladies' room. The offer seemed gentlemanly, though. It reminded me of romantic movies where a man takes a woman's arm and walks street-side, so it is he who gets the splash of manure from the passing carriages. I responded with what I believed was the most genteel response. "Sir, that is most kind."

I went to pee, and true to his word, the visit was 100% free of accosting. As I exited, I saw my bathroom guardian leaning against a wall with his arms crossed over his chest. He looked deep in contemplation, but he raised his eyes to me as I walked by. Maybe it's the sorority recruitment chair in me, but I have difficulty leaving an introduction unresolved. This man needed a sincere thanks and a proper farewell.

"Thanks again." I said. I would have said, "Have a good evening," but that's tough to do in an Emergency Room. More like, "I hope your evening is as good as it can be."

"I'm here for my brother," he replied.

"Oh, that's bad news. What brings him here tonight?"

"A bullet."

There were a few ways I could go with this and decided on what was usually the best course in life—sincerity. "Oh, my God! I am so sorry."

"Why are you sorry? You didn't do it."

"I mean, I feel bad it happened. You must be very worried for him."

"Yeah," he muttered.

"He's in the right place now. The doctors will take good care of him."

"Why are you here?"

For some unknowable reason, at this moment I deviated from the path of sincerity and made the decidedly uncool choice to try to be cool. "I'm here for my Boo."

He snickered. "Your Boo?"

"My husband."

"Car accident? "

"Liver transplant. He's a transplant patient."

He gave me a look as if he was appraising the truthfulness of my statement. It reminded me I would not want to be on the business end of his displeasure. I'd seen that look before — namely from my father, who served as an Army interrogator during the Vietnam war. I nervously began to over-explain. "There is an organ transplant center here. My husband is on the organ transplant waiting list. For a liver."

That answer seemed to satisfy.

"I sure hope your brother is okay."

"Yeah. He came through the last time."

Last time!?! I tried to hide my look of shock. "Well, my very best wishes to him...and to you."

"You too. And your...Boo," he said through a barely concealed chuckle.

I returned to Jim, but the situation had not improved.

"They come by with some drugs yet?"

"No."

"Has anyone been here since I stepped out?"

"No."

As I adjusted his pillows and piled both of our coats over him, another resident came into the room. I regurgitated my speech about his medical history and reiterated the request for medication.

"He is clearly in pain. The first doctor said there would be medication right away."

"I will look into that."

More time passed. Enter a new doctor. I regurgitated the speech and reiterated the request for medication. "Where is the pain medication they promised him?"

"We are looking into that."

New doctor then asked me another round of questions.

I kept explaining Jim was under the care of the transplant doctors in this very same hospital and Jim had been in this very same hospital earlier this week. I gently reminded him he had full access to all of Jim's records. I also reminded him he could call any of Jim's doctors on my phone right now, on speaker, to get a consultation. For all I knew, one or more of them was on the premises right now.

This doctor was treating Jim's ailment like a first-time diagnosis. He recommended Jim have a therapeutic tap. Doctors anesthetize the skin and then pierce it with a needle. This helps removes fluid from a patient's abdomen. Jim had abdominal taps back in June during his first hospital stay.

For a patient with ascites, getting tapped feels fantastic. It's like losing 20 pounds in a single day. You walk with a lighter step; you feel better. So much of the heavy discomfort goes away. However, doctors strongly advise transplant patients against getting them.

There are a few reasons for this. The big ones are:

1. possible introduction of infection, and
2. body chemistry.

As to the former: While hospitals take every precaution to make everything as germ-free as possible, they don't always win the battle. There could be dangerous bacteria on the needle or on the equipment used to do the tap. The entry wound could also get infected. It was best to avoid this possibility by skipping taps entirely.

As to the latter: Keeping Jim from tipping over the edge into liver or kidney failure meant rigorous attention to the measurement and composition of body fluids. He had just spent over a week in the hospital, where medical staff measured so much as a thimble-full of fluid going in or coming out. The doctors had worked so hard to achieve that balance, I really didn't want to upset it. Neither did Jim. He heard "tap" and started shaking his head vigorously.

"No. He does not consent to the tap."

"Well then, we can't treat him. Because we don't know what's wrong."

"I know what's wrong. He needs a new liver."

The doctor then leveled me with that withering look you give to someone who just let out a thunderous fart in church.

"What do we need to do to decrease his pain?"

"If you let me do a tap, we can find out what's wrong."

"Can you call his liver doctors first?"

"They would want me to take this step to see if there is an infection."

Finally, I asked of the day, "If you do this, will you give him pain medication?"

"Yes."

"Do it."

Jim — despite being in agony — was insistent that they take as little as possible to keep with at least half of our doctor's orders. He didn't even flinch when the needle went in.

"You have what you need. Please medicate him."

"I will send someone right away," he said as he departed with his precious sample.

Much like *"awhile," "right away"* is a relative term in a hospital. Still, this *right away* had already taken three hours. After waiting 10 minutes, I poked my head out impatiently. After another 20, a brand-new doctor came in.

"What seems to be happening with you, sir?" New New doctor asked cheerfully.

"A. Whole. Lot." I said tensely.

"Oh."

"We are waiting on pain medication."

"Did someone get your medical history?"

"Yes."

"Well...I just started my shift..."

I proceeded to explain in perfect-diction staccato Jim's entire medical history, course of treatment, social security number, and the name of every doctor with whom he had spoken, including time stamps.

"I see. Let me get someone to help ri—"

"Please don't say 'right away.' Because 'right away' is now going on eight hours."

"Okay," Third New Doctor practically ran from the room.

Another ten minutes passed, and it occurred to me I may have frightened away Jim's last hope of help tonight. Jim was silently weeping on the bed. His face was red and soaked with tears. This was already well past the point of acceptable.

The problem was I had been acting patiently and rationally in the face of crazy. Emergency Rooms are crazy places. When faced with crazy, you gotta go bigger crazy. And that's what happened.

I strutted up to the nurses' station. Two nurses were entering information into computer terminals while chatting with one another.

"Excuse me."

They continued their conversation.

"EXCUSE ME!!!"

They looked up. I now had their full attention.

"My husband requested pain medication over THREE HOURS AGO. He is WRITHING IN PAIN and he is CRYING. WE. NEED. HELP."

"I will see to that right—"

"DON'T YOU SAY, 'RIGHT AWAY' TO ME. NO ONE may SAY, 'RIGHT AWAY' TO ME." I paused and took a deep calming breath. "I would like to accompany you while we—together—find a nurse or doctor who can administer the requested pain medication to my husband IMMEDIATELY."

As she scurried around with me nipping at her heels, she quickly rallied a team together. They then swarmed Jim with a team of four attentive physicians and nurses. There were offers of extra blankets. There were soothing remarks. And — for the love of God — there was a big, beautiful, blessed needle filled with morphine going into his IV drip.

As Jim's body slackened with relief, I felt a backlash of remorse. The nurse whom I accosted stood next to me, watching all the action.

I turned to her. "I owe you an apology. You didn't cause this problem, but you solved it. Thank you."

"You said he's your husband, right?"

"Yeah."

"You were only trying to do right by him. Love gets loud sometimes."

"…And crazy."

"That too," she smiled knowingly.

The night ended about two hours and a 15-minute stretcher ride to the liver ward later, where we saw more than a few friendly faces.

The issue was unknown, but for the moment, Jim was comfortable and in good hands. After the requisite fussing with blankets, pillows, trays and chargers, it was time for my exit. I chugged the energy drink I had been saving for a *very special occasion* and prepared to take the 2 a.m. drive home. I flipped through the music on my iPhone.

Dr. Horrible:
It's a brand new me
I got no remorse
Now the water's rising
But I know the course...
It's a brand-new day.

Facebook Group
Jim's Liver Party
January 19 – Late Night Edition

TJ: "Doctors admitted Jim last night via the Emergency Room. He was in a great deal of pain. After some morphine for Jim and an endless day for the both of us, he took the now familiar ride up the elevator to the liver ward. Doctors ruled out an infection, which is very, very good news. Nevertheless, there's no real answers for what's going wrong now.

Tomorrow morning, Jim is getting an ultrasound. As a liver patient, we already know his gall bladder looks like a bag of marbles and his spleen ain't pretty. This ultrasound is to make sure nothing is, say, exploding.

In most medical cases, there would be much investigation. ("Is it your gall bladder, a kidney stone? What could it be?") With liver patients, it's more like, "You seem to be out of pain and not dead. Victory!" The end goal is transplant. Everything in the middle is noise.

A good/bad bit of news is that Jim's latest MELD is 26. The change was due to improved kidney function (lower Creatinine: Yay!), partially offset by crappier liver function. But, while he is still in the big time (MELD 25+), this could impact the 'ordering' on the transplant list. We hope not."

CHAPTER 10: JANUARY 19-30

City Hospital, Jim's Room

I visited Jim the morning after the Emergency Room extravaganza to check on him.

He didn't look great. He was the color of Mountain Dew, but he at least looked more comfortable than yesterday.

"It was all that football," I teased. "Too much excitement for you."

Jim hit me with a mock horrified expression.

"Next time you'll just need to settle for a fainting couch and a round of smelling salts."

There were lots of ins and outs all day from the doctors and nurses. Jim had become a bit of a fan favorite. If you could genetically mix a saint and a sloth, that would be a conservative estimation of Jim's level of patience. He also had the manners of Galant (of *Highlights for Children* fame) and could be a pleasant chatterbox. One nurse had even taken to calling him "Boo" — managing to sell it a whole lot better than I did.

The other thing working in his favor was that liver wards weren't specifically for transplant patients. Patients who had substance abuse issues were there, too. Several were known to be, let us say, unworthy of the title of "Boo."

There was one lady who went completely cuckoo bananas. "Where's my tray at?" echoed through the liver ward as she repeatedly screamed at the nurses. Apparently the hospital staff had bussed her dinner tray before she had finished with it. Another time we witnessed one patient checking himself out against doctor's orders.

The doctors patiently explained they thought it was best he stayed and that any departure would be against medical advice and may affect his insurance. He got them to take out his IV and then just grabbed his bag of patient belongings and trotted to the elevator, still wearing his hospital gown. I wondered if his plan was to call an Uber like that. He left behind some vape pens in the room for Jim and me, so that was super nice.

The plan was to do an ultrasound in the morning and then send Jim home around lunchtime tomorrow. The news stations predicted snow, so the timing was dreadful.

Jim's mission all day was — when someone told him he was going to be discharged — to ask, "Are you sure it will be tomorrow?" The result every time was, "Yes." Hospitals are for wellness, not for everyday living. When a hospital wants you out, they want you out. I've never been a good snow driver, so I was looking forward to this Jim pick up about as much as a tooth extraction.

Jim was oblivious to how much this snow storm was weighing on me. A thing you both simultaneously love and can't stand about those with a long-term illness is they become divorced from everyday realities. Jim's job was living. Jim had also not made dinner, changed a lightbulb, done a load of laundry, or cleaned a cat box in months.

I get that when things like walking to the bathroom feel like running a 100 meter dash, you lose perspective. I tried to remember that when — exhausted from a 16-hour day — Jim starts a text string with me about his last walk to the bathroom.

My parents, who have a sixth sense about this kind of thing, stepped in to offer family support. That afternoon they showed up on my doorstep bearing homemade spaghetti sauce and meatballs (because we're from New Jersey) and a family-sized bottle of bourbon. Then they sat down with me and we developed our plan of attack.

The first order of business was to get prepared. Dad made sure the snowblower was tanked up while I gathered all the usual stuff we would need for a hospital discharge, including winter weather gear for Jim.

The next order of business was laying out our respective roles.

Dad would be the driver. My father was a retired corporate attorney. He also has a quiet badass streak. He is kind and smart and funny, but also was not the type of guy you trifle with. I'd like to say that it was his time in the Army that taught him all he needed to know about driving in hazardous conditions. The truthful answer is my dad did a lot of driving, having played in traveling bands for the better part of his seven decades — high school bands, party bands, college bands, wedding bands — you name it. New Jersey party people give zero fucks about the weather when they want to dance to and throw back some cocktails. Ever hear the phrase, "And the band played on..."? They were probably talking about my dad playing a New Jersey wedding during a hurricane.

The point being, my father had, for many years, driven trucks filled with expensive equipment through whatever monsoon, snowstorm or general calamity failed to keep bar goers away. He wasn't *Ice Road Truckers* material, but he was as close as you could get in a Toyota.

My role was to be the Jim wrangler. Finally, Mom would manage things on the home-front and serve as the second-shift Jim wrangler after our arrival home.

Between the three of us — we could do this.

Our House, Next Day

I got up at my usual time these days — about 4 a.m. — to get in a few hours of work before we set off.

The hospital said discharge would be around 9 a.m. This was early for them. The usual discharge time was the super-convenient time of 11 a.m. However, we figured the doctors and nurses who worked there were concerned about snow, too, and wanted to front-load the day.

Dad and I were caffeinated by 7:30 a.m. and in the car by 7:45 a.m. The snow started soon after we got on the road. It was that kind of snow that comes in those fat, pillowy flakes.

We immediately knew the answer to the seminal New Jersey question: *Will it stick?*

The answer: *Abso-freaking-lutely.*

As we pulled into the hospital, there was a good inch-plus on the ground. I walked Dad through the *park here's, walk here's* and *turn there's.* I was a veteran visitor at this point.

When we got to Jim's room, we were pleased to find out he had already received the ultrasound results (which were as predicted) and had green lights to go from all the necessaries. The final checkpoint was one of the liver doctors.

Since the general tone of the daily doctors' consults involved comments like "healthy enough" and "not sure what else we can do," we were pretty sure the final discharge order would come quickly and we could get the proverbial show on the road.

I did my routine of going around the room and helping Jim pack. I suggested he get dressed too, but as he reminded me, "Sometimes they like to poke at the belly to test me for doneness!"

With gown on and bags packed, it was now a waiting game.

The first hour of waiting was what one might expect. Dad and I spent most of the time looking out the window and watching the city transform into the North Pole.

Then the second hour went by.

Dad suggested I make quiet overtures to the hospital staff about moving things along. Some of these people would soon have their hands in Jim's abdomen, however, and I didn't the very people with the power to replace my husband's failing liver with a similarly proportioned turnip to label me a troublesome spouse.

I was also hip to the fact that we were in a hospital. While Jim was taking a brisk walk to the death race finish line, others were zooming down the fast lane. The latter needed doctor's intervention. If I had to look at LOL cats on my iPhone while they saved someone's life, so be it.

At hour three, the doctor finally made his appearance.

At this point, we estimated there was more than half a foot of snow on the ground. My father and I were edgy, but I still put on my very best 20,000-watt smile. "I hope you did okay, getting here in the snow!" I greeted him.

"Oh, it's snowing?" He asked, looking out of the giant window in front of him. "I didn't really notice."

Okay. What?

This was a doctor Jim had not seen before, but I remembered his picture. He was the surgeon who ran the liver transplant practice.

You got a new team of doctors every time you "graduated" in the program. For a pre-transplant patient like Jim, you would see a rotating team of doctors (charged with keeping you alive) and surgeons (charged with getting the new organ in and working well). This gentleman helped to pioneer the program and now worked with the post-transplant patients — two years or more after transplant. Since that was nothing but a hoped-for dream for us at this point, it was no surprise we had not met him before.

The doctor flipped through Jim's mountain of paperwork without so much as glancing up at us. So much for poking the belly.

What you have to understand is that the liver ward was a warm and friendly place for us. Over the course of the past seven months, we had gotten to know the team well — doctors, nurses and surgeons. I knew who had a fondness for shoe shopping and which doctor had recently published a book of poetry (that yes; we bought on Amazon). This doctor's non-verbal approach immediately made me think we'd somehow screwed up.

"It must be a busy time for you and the team. Any transplants this week?" I chimed in cheerfully.

"No." He responded, not looking up.

This was weird, too. Transplants brought everyone to life on this team. While they could never share patient details, the doctors and surgeons were always happy to share stuff like, "We had a long one last night, but the patient is doing great!"

Finally, the doctor lifted his head and said, "I'd like to keep him at least another day. Come back tomorrow." With no further explanation he began to head toward the door.

"May I ask why the extension?" I practically shouted after him.

"His ammonia. It's elevated. I'd like to observe him."

"His ammonia has already been pretty high for a while now."

"Yes."

"He's quite lucid."

"Sure."

"I'm not sure if we can get here tomorrow," I said lamely.

That was when the doctor hit me with his first smile of the day. "You'll figure something out."

As the doctor left, I turned to Jim. "Has he talked to you? Like, at all? Any time today or yesterday?"

"No, he hasn't."

Now, honestly, I wasn't knocking the doctor for being unfriendly. This discussion was important.

Liver patients have elevated levels of ammonia. It causes a condition called Hepatic Encephalopathy or HE. At high levels of ammonia, patients can begin to have cognitive difficulties and mood challenges. A less charitable way of saying it would be: They go Cuckoo Bananas. 70% of cirrhosis patients get it. For some, it can be debilitating.

Jim was a unique case in that his levels were high enough to indicate he *could* exhibit symptoms of HE. Jim just didn't. For reasons unknown, it didn't seem to impact Jim the way it did other patients. Jim was as placid as a lake on a windless day. He could speak to you— at length, in detail, and with clarity—on a wide range of subjects. Sometimes until your ears bled. I would argue that Jim could have easily won the hospital's trivia tournament. (Well, they didn't actually have a trivia tournament, but there ought to have been one because hospitals are pretty boring places.)The point is that if you *actually spoke* to Jim, you'd realize in under 60 seconds he readily demonstrated the logic of a college professor and the emotional intelligence of Deepak Chopra.

In short: This doctor just didn't know my Boo.

When Dining Services walked in with a lunch tray, we knew it was our cue to exit.

City, On the Road

We decided to take most of the stuff home and leave Jim with the barest essentials. Our hope was to make a hasty exit tomorrow.

Dad and I hightailed it to the car — which more accurately involved us trudging through growing drifts.

Now, when one is going on a road trip, it's ideal if you share the same general vibe as your travel partner. Dad and I were both in a Fuck this shit mood, characterized by a sense of purpose, and Level 10 gallows humor. The latter was in top form during the hour-plus it took us to even turn out of the parking garage.

My Midwestern friends would snicker, and my Canadian friends would guffaw, but anything above two inches and New Jersey basically breaks. This was also a busy city with an under-funded snow removal budget. Basically, there was an ice-cold hot mess on our hands.

These were whiteout conditions — where everything was the same color and you kept running your windshield blades with increasingly limited visibility. It was the equivalent of driving through city streets while staring through a periscope lens.

We inched down the streets. Despite the dreadful weather conditions, this was still a pedestrian city. So, we had to keep our eyes out for the errant local dashing across the street to the bodega. At one point, we contemplated finding a nearby place to stay the night. All the area hotels were off the main highway, though. That wouldn't do us any good.

There were also very few places to pull over and wait it out. The sections of the city we had to drive through to get to the hospital were tightly clustered collections of homes and apartments on streets so narrow you could barely get your car through the parked cars on both sides.

No, we were right and truly screwed and just had to make do for the time being, inch by frozen inch. I started by making idle chatter, but as the time wore on and the snow bore down, we flicked on the music instead. I scrolled through the selections and put on Peter Allen, one of my mom's favorites, because if Dad and I did wind up dying in a car wreck, the newspaper would then be obliged to write a story titled, "No Go to Rio — Father and daughter's snowy hospital errand ends in tragic accident to musical accompaniment of Australian-born singer-songwriter."

"You should give Mom an update," my dad said, keeping eyes firmly on the road.

"Good idea."

I figured a call on speaker might be too distracting. While Dad was a master at presenting the "placid and steady Dad face," I could see he was white knuckling the wheel. Instead, I started a text string and read Dad the highlights. I pictured Mom sitting in my kitchen in a thick bathrobe, cell phone flat on my kitchen table while she poked at it with her stylus. My mom, among her many wonderful features, has the fingernails of an elegantly groomed mountain lion. A proud Luddite, she'd only recently started texting. This was as good an occasion as any to practice.

Me: Hey, Mom.
Mom: Are you on the road now? [Eek Face Emoji]
Me: Yes. Driving home now.
Mom: How are the roads?

"She's asking about the drive."
"She'll be worried." Dad responded.
"Should I go vague on this?"
"Yup."

Me: It's slow going.
Mom: When do you think you'll be home?
Me: Not sure yet. We can give you a better ETA a little later.

Mom: (Insert 20 rapid-fire questions about road safety, our safety, relative level of hunger, access to fluids, access to blankets, and meteorological conditions.)

The truth started oozing out of me. You can't ever maintain vagueness with a worried New Jersey mother. Finally, I seemed to satisfy her barrage of questions.

Me: See you when we see you.
Mom: Drive safe. LOL.

I stared at my screen, a bit puzzled. "So, Mom ends it with, 'Drive Safe. LOL.'"

"Are you serious?"

"Yes. Drive Safe. LOL."

"LOL? That's like going, 'Sorry, I just ran over your dog. HA-HA HAAAAA!!!'"

"Or 'It's Cancer. Stage 4. HA-HA HAAAAA!!!'"

We continued this riff for the next three hours.

When we're about a half an hour away from home, I sent Mom another update.

Me: Almost home.
Mom: Okay. See you soon. LOL.

Dad and I laughed so hard I nearly peed myself.

When we pulled into the driveway exhausted and hungry and walked in the front door, greeted by the aroma of homemade spaghetti sauce and garlic bread.

While Mom plated the eats, Dad and I made a beeline to the bourbon, pouring ourselves a good 4+ fingers each.

"I have been a wreck worrying about you guys," my mom said.

"Well, you'd never know that," I laughed.

"What? Why?"

Dad and I exchanged baffled looks.

"What do you think LOL means?" My dad finally asked.

"Lots of Love. Why?"

Dad and I took one more look at each other and laughed until our sides hurt.

Facebook Group
Jim's Liver Party
February 21

TJ: "Wanted to give everybody an update on Jim's health. His MELD score has decreased to a 21 after the high of 28 when he started having kidney problems. He just sort of feels icky — incomparably tired, some gastrointestinal issues, etc. But he is comfortable, and for the past few days, enjoyed a visit with Jay! Some of Jim's test scores showed the potential for some internal bleeding, so I'm taking him for an endoscopy with Dr. Kenney on Thursday. He is being well looked after and in good spirit, which is not too shabby for a guy who really needs a freaking liver. Sending love and hugs!"

Facebook Group
Jim's Liver Party
February 24

TJ: "Bit of a health setback over the weekend. Jim was in a lot of pain. Eager to avoid another Emergency Room visit, Jim took meds and soldiered on through. Since liver patients metabolize drugs differently than healthier folks, he spent most of Sunday in a fog. Upside? Advised him it's probably as close to drunk as he's been in a good long while. Endoscopy on for this week. He has an issue with internal bleeding. Doctor doesn't seem too concerned. However, this is how they're going to figure out what's going on. In the meantime, he's just dog tired. I suppose that's why I don't feel badly making him watch the season finale of Downton Abbey with me tonight. It will give him ample opportunity for a much-needed nap."

CHAPTER 11: FEBRUARY & EARLY MARCH

Our House, Living Room

Jim's friend Jay, who usually worked abroad, stayed with us for a few days during his trip back to the U.S. Jay needed a rest and Jim had no other options but to rest, so the two spent many hours sitting in front of the TV together.

I was trying to keep things light on social media, but the at-home situation was pretty rough. Jim was sleeping even more than before. He was uncomfortable. He was always out of breath. The only food he could stomach was fruit popsicles, but it became increasingly difficult to get him to even eat that.

His health was increasingly fragile, and I was working from home as often as I could to care for him. When doctors suspected Jim may have internal bleeding, I planned to take the day off of work to get him over to Dr. Kenney to do an endoscopy. They would put Jim under general anesthesia and put a camera down his throat to check out his digestive tract and perhaps find the cause of the bleeding.

For the healthy person, an endoscopy is a minor inconvenience. For the unwell person, an endoscopy is an all-day health extravaganza.

If I was being really honest with myself, I felt a good bit of crankiness. I didn't want to take him for this test. I was already taking him for a lot of tests and general poking every week. Thursdays were doctor visits. Fridays were blood tests. This was a Wednesday. This was usually the day I would spend trying to do all the things I couldn't do on Thursday and Friday. Losing another day this week meant working all weekend. I didn't mind working all weekend, but then I couldn't get my weekend chores done.

On the upside, the appointment was local, with Dr. Kenney. We really liked him, and he was really, really good at his job. I just didn't want to see him today.

I heard Jim talking on the phone while I was in the other room and investigated. "Honey, what's up?" I asked when the call ended.

"Doctor Kenney called. He wants to cancel the procedure today. He said something is up with my blood levels. He's calling Doctor Attia."

"It's probably not a big deal, right?"

"This sucks. I needed to get this done."

"Yes, and I know."

There was at least a small possibility this really wasn't a big deal. If you showed your average family physician Jim's chart, she would probably go, "How is this guy not dead!?!" Show the same chart to a doctor dealing with end stage liver disease, she'd go, "Keep him hydrated and see you next week." While Dr. Kenney was a gastroenterologist, he dealt in wellness. Instinct said this could be a matter of adjusting procedures for a transplant patient. For example: Since Jim's metabolism was now that of a turtle on a fist full of Quaaludes, Dr. Kenney may have had some genuine concerns about anesthesia.

Jim's phone lit up. It was Dr. Attia calling. *This* was not good. He put her on speaker.

She kicked it off with her normal pleasantries. We loved Dr. Attia. Besides her being a brilliant physician, she was sunshine embodied.

"Jim, we're going to need to get you to the hospital."

"What's wrong?"

"Dr. Kenney didn't like what he was seeing on your blood test and reached out to me. He was concerned, and I agree with him."

"So, no endoscopy."

"No endoscopy."

"So, we'll see you tomorrow then, I guess?" Jim's regular appointment with her was on Thursdays.

Dr. Attia sighed deeply then, and the whole world seemed to get heavier. "I'm really sorry, Jim, but you have to come to the hospital now."

"Okay." For the first time, in a very long time, Jim started to lose it. Big, fat tears ran down his cheeks.

"Jim, are you there?"

He signaled for me to talk.

"Dr. Attia, it's TJ. I heard what you said, and I'll get him up there. Does this look like an admission thing?"

"I think it does. I'm going to have the Admissions folks reach out to you."

"No Emergency Room. That's like Christmas!"

Dr. Attia laughed. "I like your optimism. We'll see you guys soon, okay?"

"Got it."

"Jim, stay strong. We're here to take good care of you."

My community theater background and years as a sorority recruitment chair had an immediate and tangible impact on my personal life in this moment. It was time to forget about being grumpy. I had a sad, dying man next to me. It was my mission to make this the most fun hospital trip ever.

"We're going to get this sorted, okay? And, hey, your go-bag is already packed!"

"I don't know how much longer I can do this."

"I know."

"I am just so, so, so fucking tired."

"This is just another setback. But you've dealt with this before. Keep your eyes on the prize!"

Admission called right away. I explained Jim's situation, saying I just didn't think he could take waiting hours up there for a bed. I claimed it was because of physical discomfort — ascites, exhaustion, sitting in those chairs. That was all true, but the bigger reason was that I didn't think his soul could take it. I had the distinct feeling that six hours in the Admission waiting room would break my guy.

They agreed to let Jim wait in comfort at home. When it looked as if a bed would be available, they would call us, and we promised to get in the car ASAP.

I sat Jim in front of the living room TV while I raced around to do all of the necessaries. One never knew how long they'd be in the hospital. I left the cats enough food for a feast and gathered all of our stuff.

Two hours later, we got the call and headed up. True to their word, he for once didn't have to wait for a bed.

City Hospital, Jim's Room

I took the lead on the admission questions, medical history, and drug stuff because Jim was uncharacteristically despondent and a little out of it. Who could blame him? He'd spent the better part of a month in the hospital and his February MELD scores made a liver transplant an unlikely short-term possibility.

I kept Jim's struggles off his/my main Facebook feeds, instead posting occasional updates to the small Jim's Liver Party group. Today, I made an exception. I posted something to Jim's and my pages about his hospital stay, asking people to post fun memes, silly stories, or anything to distract him. I passed the time by handing him my phone to look at the pictures or reading him some funny posts. He would very occasionally crack a smile, I think mostly to appease me. Today was not a good day.

Dr. Laghari, another one of our favorite doctors, finally walked into the room a couple hours later. He was a newer physician but continued to show wisdom, professionalism and passion beyond his years.

"How are you doing tonight, Jim?" He asked brightly.

"Not so good. You tell me."

He dove into the diagnosis. "Jim, your sodium levels are very, very low, as is your white count. We need to do some things to get those up, okay?"

Jim nodded and looked out the window. Dr. Laghari gave him a long look.

"Jim has been a little, um, sad today," I said.

"I can imagine. I know this has been a long road for him. And for you."

"May I speak with you privately a moment?"

"Let's head to the hallway."

We left Jim's room and walked a few feet down the hall.

"How serious is this? What's going on now?"

"I would say this is quite serious. The issue here is really his salt. It's dangerously low. That's why your other doctor called off the procedure. Let me ask...does he seem like himself today?"

"No. No, he doesn't. Very sad. Kind of out of it."

Dr. Laghari nodded. "We're going to do everything we can right now to rebalance everything in his system. But, his condition is...delicate. We must keep a very close watch on him for the next 12 hours. This is quite serious."

"Are you saying he might not make it...to transplant?"

"Well...know that we're going to do our absolute best to get him there."

"What can I do?"

"Keep him awake and engaged. Keep his spirits up. Let us do our work to help him."

"Okay."

"You're a very strong supporter. You've got this."

I don't got this.

I don't got this at all.

I was at the polar opposite of *got this*.

I felt like a total poser. I didn't know what I was doing. I was a lady who couldn't balance a checkbook. I forgot birthdays. I never remembered to change the oil in my car. I was now responsible for the survival of another human being. Was I *really* up for this?

No, I was not.

Still, I sure was going to try. What do you talk about with someone in the hospital who is freezing in a drafty room, who is tired beyond measure, and was just told not to buy any green bananas?

It needed to be a topic so tantalizing to Jim, he couldn't help but get excited and insist on sharing his myriad of opinions.

Then it came to me.

Le Bernardin.

Le Bernardin was a French restaurant specializing in truly outstanding fish. Eric Ripert is its famous chef. Justo Thomas is the fish butcher who is so phenomenally precise that they have to bring on three people to replace him whenever he takes a well-deserved vacation. Anthony Bourdain was a devoted fan. It has won virtually every culinary award. You needed reservations months in advance. It was a NYC institution.

Jim and I had never been. But it's something that would pop up in conversation occasionally. Jim and I had been lucky enough to dine in some great places around the world, but this one — this relatively local one — continued to elude us. Well, tonight it might very well save his life.

My opening gambit: "Well, Jim. You just have to get past this shit so we can go to *Le Bernardin*."

"What?"

"You can't go there like this." I gestured to his hospital gown and general girth. "We must get you a nice, new suit."

"A suit?" He asked dazedly.

"Yes. So, you can wear it to *Le Bernardin*. I'm guessing after the transplant you'll be all svelte, so we can order you something bespoke if you'd like. But back to dinner. What are you going to order?"

"Tonight?"

"No, not tonight. We're clearly very busy tonight." I gestured around the room. "But another night. What are you going to order?"

"Where?"

"*Le Bernardin*. What are you doing to get at *Le Bernardin*?"

He looked at my face, and his eyes focused. *"Oysters. I want oysters."*

I smiled and nodded at him. "I can picture you slurping them while I smell the beautiful flowers."

"One does not *slurp* at *Le Bernardin*." He paused, then looked at me. I had him. "What are you having?"

Thus began an all-night conversation about a restaurant where he would likely never get to eat. We talked about our waiter. We debated if he would truly be French or a Brooklyn actor acting French. We never quite resolved our answers on that one.

We talked about the seating. We both agreed we wouldn't be sufficiently famous to be seated by the window, but that we would ask and take our chances.

We would do the chef's menu versus a la carte. The Chef is one of the best in the world. We would naturally trust his judgement.

We talked through every culinary possibility, including a thorough dissection of the assumed breadbasket.

As the hours got smaller, we talked on—while the doctors and nurses came in and out of the room doing the work of keeping him around.

We had an entire meal over the course of the night, talking about every nuance of the place. Then, in the morning, we got the best possible news: Jim had turned a corner. The war was still on, but this battle had been won.

As I left him at the hospital that morning to head into work, I felt full. Full of hope. Full of possibilities.

Le Bernardin had become our unlikely battle cry. Because he still had a whole lot of living to do. So, yes. He would get past this shit.

We would get past this shit.

One day, we would have that meal.

Just not today.

Facebook Group
Jim's Liver Party
February 27

TJ: "Back at the hospital with Jim this afternoon. While he is getting some treatments, let me get you up to speed...*Here is the story: Jim's MELD is now 27. Bilirubin and INR are high. The biggest problem, though, is the salt, which remains dangerously low. (I know: Irony! Because he can't eat any!) Doctors now have to watch the kidneys very, very carefully. Adjusting the salt too fast will send them into distress, which is not a good thing. Doctor described this as a bit of a delicate time and wants to keep Jim here until they have it under control. This is not a 'get out today' style ailment. Jim got to rest last night (morphine, baby!) and seems to respond well to albumin infusions. But, as you imagine, this whole extravaganza is wearing on him. On the upside, Jim's next-door neighbor apparently got the word today that he is being discharged. Upon hearing the news, he boisterously yelled, 'I'm gettin' out, bitches!!!' In a few days, one hopes Jim will say the same."*

Facebook Group
Jim's Liver Party
February 28

TJ: *"Salt is a little better today. (Up to 121 vs low of 117.) Doctors are pleased with this progress. Ascites kicking in again. Blood counts are not good, so Jim needs a transfusion. (His first!) Getting that this afternoon. He is feeling a bit weak and spacey but is eating well. (He totally ate an entire tray of food today! It's the first time he has done this in a very long time. He clearly prefers the hospital cooking to mine.) Walked a few steps today. It pleased nurses that Jim his exercise on. Jim continues to be the darling of his ward."*

Reagan's House

Jim was becoming less and less himself.

He'd started to lose interest in the news, his mainstay. He also started getting confused and referring to people by the wrong names — close, but wrong. Our friend Reagan became Renee. Jay became John.

Meanwhile, I was quietly fading.

I had three focus areas:

1. Jim: Each day this involved about three hours in the car, three-to-six hours at the hospital, and two hours of general health management (prescriptions, doctor calls, filling out forms).
2. Work: Because someone had to ensure we had this swell thing called health insurance, I spent about five hours a day in the office and then handled about two hours of email in the early morning and another two hours late at night.
3. Chores: Salt-free food didn't buy or prepare itself and clothes didn't wash themselves, so this took up the rest of the time I wasn't asleep.

I wasn't eating much because the thought of cooking for myself was too daunting. Plus, if I sat still for a full ten minutes, I would fall asleep. Water for pasta takes about fifteen minutes to boil, so I was in serious risk of burning the house down.

For a while I had focused on using up things Jim could no longer. (Hello, scotch!) There was always that random box of Saltines tucked to the back of the cabinet or Stouffer's frozen pizza. When I found a salty treasure, I did my best not to eat it in front of him.

Mom would stock my freezer. Those meals became my big Saturday night treats. I would get home from the hospital in the early evening, nuke myself some pot roast, and savor every bite before I passed out on the couch.

Beyond that, I was a dietary wasteland.

At eight o'clock on a Friday night, when a balanced meal seemed entirely out of reach, my phone lit up with a text from Reagan. Reagan is the queen of texting. She is very stream-of-consciousness about it. One minute I will get a text asking about movies and the next is sending me a link *to a new shower curtain she urges me to buy.*

Reagan: Have you eaten yet?
Me: No. About to drive home from the hospital.
Reagan: Stop here on the way. I will feed you.
Me: But it will be, like, 9:30 at night.
Reagan: COME. HERE.

I arrived at 9:47 p.m. She answered the door in her jammies. I protested that it was too late, but she shuffled me right into her kitchen and plopped me in a chair. She set a glass next to me.

"It's a gin and tonic," she said before I could ask. "Drink it."

"You having one too?"

"Of course I am." She pulled something that smelled delicious out of the microwave. "It's beef bourguignon. Eat it." She had put enough food on my plate to feed a high school football team.

"Wow. Thank you."

"No wow. It's leftovers. But they're good."

I tucked into my beef, which was insanely good.

"Okay, now tell me everything."

Gin, beef and human kindness have a way of making people open up.

"I think Jim is going to die."

The words spilled out of me. It was the first time I'd ever said it out loud. Even to say it felt like blasphemy. Your job as a transplant caregiver was to be unfailingly optimistic.

Rationally, I always knew this was a possibility. People on the transplant waiting list die every day. I just wasn't ready for Jim to be one of them. It was a possibility I'd never let myself truly consider. But now it was here, right in front of me.

Reagan didn't give me platitudes. Instead, she refilled my glass and let me talk.

"Thank you. For listening," I said over an hour later.

"Of course."

"Just don't tell anyone, okay? Especially Jim. Don't tell people I was worried about...about...him not getting the transplant."

"You? Being a human being with genuine worries? I will be sure to keep that to myself."

Our House, Front Door

At 7:55 a.m. the next morning, my doorbell rang. Mitch was standing on my doorstep.

A few days earlier he'd offered to drive me up to the hospital. I'd politely refused because Saturdays were usually all-day hospital extravaganzas. That's just a lot to ask someone to commit to — especially someone whose kids are in traveling sports.

But he *had* slyly inquired about what time I usually left ("a little after eight") and took it upon himself to just show up so I couldn't refuse. It embarrassed me. My caregiver role had been a solo thing from the start. When other people entered the mix, I always felt as if I had to keep them happy, and that stressed me out. I didn't want to have to make the hospital fun today.

"Let's get some coffee." He said as we hit the road.

We stopped at Wawa and as we pulled into a spot he said, "You know, you can let people help you."

Always right to the point, this guy.

"I know that."

"I know you *know* that, but I don't think you *get* that."

I give him a withering look.

"You're about to say something funny or redirect the conversation, but you don't have to entertain me."

Mind reader?

We got back in the car and I started blowing on my too-hot coffee. I was keen to chug it. I asked Mitch about work and about his family. He had lots to say on both subjects and settling back to just listen was nice. Finally, we settled into comfortable silence, then: "So how is he really?"

"Not good, Mitch. Not at all good."

He did that move now where you take a good long pause before asking another question. It's a great tactic. Keep them talking. I didn't think I would fall for it, but of course I did.

"I just don't know if he's going to get a transplant."

Wow, I was seriously on a roll.

"He may be too sick to get one."

"But, isn't that the point?"

"What?"

"He's gotta be really sick to get one."

"Yes."

"And he's really sick."

"Yes?"

"Which means he is going to get one."

"I admire your faith."

"You seem to have lost yours."

I was about to go on the defensive, but I settled into silence and let that sink in.

Maybe I had?

I think maybe I had pictured something a little more Hollywood, where everyone was well-moisturized, and the news came about a transplant during the second part of a "very special episode."

So much of our lives had become about trying to extend his life. It was an exhausting gamble on a bet that more and more I realized we could lose.

First his mom passed. Then, it was the cirrhosis diagnosis. Then, it was all about qualifying for transplant. Then, it was the endless doctor visits, blood tests, hospital stays, drives, anxious moments. Still, Jim was wasting away before my eyes.

Would he forget my name next?

When we got to the hospital, Mitch walked in like he owned the place. It's a quality of his I've always envied—to look at home anywhere. Mitch was active in politics, so he had that ability to connect with pretty much everyone he met.

I had texted Jim on the way that Mitch was coming up with me. For Jim, this was a big deal. Visitors were few and far between because the hospital was a pretty long haul for friends and family.

Mitch sat in a chair next to Jim's bed and immediately started hitting Jim with questions while I fiddled with the things visiting spouses at the hospital always fiddle with—bed cover smoothing, general cleaning.

"I see you got your own room. How did you get to be so fancy?"

"No clue. But, not too bad, huh?"

This was something I had always speculated about. I knew my medical insurance was good, but not "room by yourself" good. During Jim's first stay he'd had a roommate who was, it could charitably be said, not close friends with either human niceties or reality. This roommate would regularly page staff members throughout the night and loudly berate them, which did not make for peaceful slumber. Jim tried just to settle back and take in the show, but not sleeping for two straight days is not particularly healing. Right after that, they moved him to a private room, and he had been in one ever since. I was convinced the staff had tagged their darling Jim as an Ebola patient or similar to guarantee him solitude.

Mitch asked Jim about the food, the bed linens, the entertainment choices.

As doctors and nurses came in and out, Mitch didn't appear to want to leave the room and Jim seemed to enjoy having him there — especially with Mitch's running commentary. Mitch had never been there before, and it was neat to hear his first-timer observations. They were both bantering with everyone coming in the door and Jim's room turned into a party zone.

The surgical team and a supporting cast of interns stopped in once a day to check Jim for surgical readiness. This was the test he always had to pass. I knew Dr. Fletcher was on duty that day. I had never met him before, but I knew him by reputation — exceptionally competent, kind, but with a serious temperament.

As the examination began, I whispered, "Mitch, we have to be quiet for this one."

"Can I watch?"

"Sure. But, no talking, okay? Jim really needs to focus. These are the surgical folks."

Jim seemed quite lucid today, but I didn't want to take our chances. He needed to give these folks his full attention.

As Dr. Fletcher began, I couldn't hear a single word he said. He spoke in a whisper so barely audible I was not sure bats could hear it.

Dr: Fletcher: (Says something to Jim.)

"Pretty good."

Dr: Fletcher: (Says something else.)

"Still a bit of trouble moving around. But okay."

Dr. Fletcher: (Turns to face his students and talks to them. They are furiously taking notes.)

Mitch and I were now leaning over to hear. I felt like I was about a foot from this man's face. What the hell were these junior doctors writing?

Dr. Fletcher: (Asks Jim something else.)
"So-so."
Dr. Fletcher: (Frowns and explains something else to Interns. Asks Jim another question.)
"Oh, this is my wife, TJ, and my friend Mitch."
Dr. Fletcher: (Smiles and says something.)

At a complete and total loss, I went with a generic, "Nice to meet you. Thank you for taking such good care of Jim."
"Honey, he asked where we live."
"Oh, near New Brunswick." Then I raised my voice louder and repeated, "NEW. BRUNSWICK."
Jim, doctor and the team laughed.
"I think we all heard you just fine."
Dr. Fletcher: (Says something else.)
"Honey, could you and Mitch leave for a second?"
"Is everything okay?"
"Dr. Fletcher just asked if you could step out so he can do a physical exam."
"Oh, gotcha. We'll be right outside."
I stepped outside with Mitch.
"What the fuck was that?" Mitch said as the door closed behind us.
"Oh, thank God! I thought I was the only one!"
"And what are they writing on their notepads?"
"I. KNOW!!!"
"You can come back in now!" Jim shouted through the door.
We come back in the room to more of the same.

Dr Fletcher: (Talks to Jim and to the Interns. They are all smiles.)

Intern: (Turns to Dr. Fletcher and asks an inaudible question.)
Dr. Fletcher: (Answers her and then suggests she ask a question of Jim.)
Intern: (Says God-knows-what to Jim.)
"The original diagnosis was NASH."
Intern: (Nods and thanks him.)
Dr. Fletcher: (Says something to Jim, and me, and Mitch. Then he seems to wait for a reaction. I've got nothing.)
"That's really good news. Thank you!" Jim said.
"Thank you!" Mitch and I responded in unison.
The team filed out.
"Honey, could you, like, hear him?"
"Barely," Jim laughed. "But I can if I really focus. I forgot you haven't met him before."
"What did he say?"
"If a liver arrived today, they would transplant me."
"See? That's good news."
"I think you're going to get a transplant this week," Mitch said.
"What makes you say that?" Jim asked.
"Just a feeling, I guess?"
"Okay. What day, then?" I challenged him.
"Tuesday."
"Well, Tuesday it is then. I will order the confetti cannon. Jim, clear your schedule!"

Facebook Group
Jim's Liver Party
March 2

TJ: "Wrapping up some stuff at home this morning before I head to the hospital. Wanted to give you the scoop... Jim's still in hospital (as I'm sure you have already guessed). No talk of a discharge date yet.

"He's at *MELD 29 for the second day in a row. They're trying to find a magical balance that gets his salt up, his ascites down (primarily managed by diuretics), and keeps his kidneys happy. (This is akin to tap dancing on a* balance beam while wearing a blindfold. This also explains why liver and kidney doctors deservedly make a lot of money.) Today the salt is 126. Huzzah! They'd like to get that as close to 130 as possible. Jim is on his second day of fluid restriction. In the middle of last night, they reintroduced diuretics* following multiple blood transfusions. The aim is for him to pee his brains out today and see if the kidneys get cranky.

"*I found myself swapping the word 'dianetics' for the word 'diuretics' the other day. I believe the hospital staff assumes I am dopey and/or a closet Scientologist.

"The transplant surgical team looked at him again yesterday. We were potentially in a situation where Jim needs a transplant to get well but is too unwell to receive a transplant. (Yes, I wrote that correctly.) I'm pleased to say that the surgeons green-lighted him for surgery again, if offered a liver. (Yes, like a marriage proposal. Patients get a "liver offer." No, I am not making that up.)"

City Hospital, Jim's Room

I headed up to the hospital again.

The doctors have been giving giving Jim blood transfusions. The medical protocol required Jim to first lie down, then sit, and then stand, which exhausted him. The transfusions took a long time because anything involving Jim and fluids is complicated.

Jim was also peeing his brains out. I think we were both quietly glad that he didn't have visitors today. Pee bottles and a little extra help from the wife got him through the worst of it.

"Funny what Mitch said about Tuesday." Jim said as he settled back into his bed.

"Oh, you know how he is with his predictions."

"Would be really nice though, right?"

"Yeah, yeah it would."

CHAPTER 12: MARCH 4

My Office

6:45 a.m.

The ground was still slippery from fresh snow, so I had to shuffle my way into the office. I was usually the first one in, so I quickly touched my security tag to the pad, opened the door and shut off the alarm.

Tuesdays were my days for one-on-one calls and meetings with my team members who we had spread throughout North America and Europe. I looked forward to these calls because they were always a bit of an adventure. Designed to be open-ended, they would all bring a list of stuff they wanted to discuss or sometimes just a general topic on which they wanted some input or guidance. Some wanted coaching. Some wanted affirmation. Some just wanted to catch up.

I adjusted my schedule so I would have conference calls straight through until noon. I left the afternoon clear to accommodate a hospital discharge.

I scheduled my first call for 8 a.m. I tackled about an hour of emails until then.

10:30 a.m.

The meetings progressed smoothly and without much drama and blessedly few action items. Jim managed things at the hospital by keeping me up-to-date with text updates.

Jim: Looks like discharge today.

Me: Yep. I'm all good to come get you when the hospital gives me the green light.

Jim: It will be good to be home. I miss you and the cats.
Me: Love you. See you later.

I was quietly sweating this discharge. Jim's health was now officially "delicate." He was very unsteady on his feet. His weight threw off his gait, he weighed around 350 pounds, much of it fluid. He would sometimes get dizzy upon standing. Getting to the bathroom was difficult and evacuating his bladder sometimes impossible. Jim even spent one sleepless night getting out of bed every 15 minutes trying desperately to pee. Nothing would come, but a painful urge to pee would not let him rest.

He rarely needed much help, but when he needed it, he needed it right away—a hand up out of a chair, water, some pills.

We had officially reached the point where Jim could not be alone anymore. My plan was to get him home from the hospital today and then work from home tomorrow while I figured out a longer-term plan.

This was all daunting, but achievable. It was just another thing on the to-do list.

11 a.m.

I got on my weekly call with Milly and she talked me through her proposed website changes. She walked me through the mockups and I asked questions. She had done some really nice work.

My cell phone rang. It was the hospital. I hit *Decline.*

"You need to get that?" Milly asked.

"No. It can wait."

I had texted Jim not twenty minutes ago. He sounded all good, or as "all good" as one can be when you're nearly dead. I needed to focus on work; I would see him in a little over two hours.

Sometimes the hospital called to confirm discharge information. I always thought it was their quiet of way of checking, "So, you'll really be here, right?" In Liver Land, patients were not always at their personal best. Resulting conditions, like hepatic encephalopathy, could turn them into loose cannons. I know of at least one patient who had been left in the dust by a family member or friend who was exhausted or overwhelmed.

By this point, Jim was a hospital frequent flyer. The nurses and doctors knew I was good for a ride home. They could wait another fifteen minutes for me to confirm, and wouldn't I look like a shining star when I called them from the car while on my way up to pick him up?

My other office line rang. I ignored it. My cell phone rang. Again. From the hospital. Again.

Were they really that worried I was going to flake out on picking him up?

"Milly, someone really needs to talk to me. Would you mind holding on for a second while I grab this?"

"No problem."

I picked up my cell phone. "This is TJ Condon. How can I help you?"

"Hi TJ, it's Madeline. From the hospital."

My blood ran cold. This was not good. Madeline was a nurse in the liver center. If she was calling, something must be wrong.

"Is Jim...okay? I thought he was fine. He is supposed to be discharged tod—"

"TJ, we found a match." Madeline said, cutting me off.

I'm not sure how much time passed before I responded, "Excuse me. Can you say that again...please? I... I am not sure I... heard you correctly."

"We think we found a match."

I had been on my feet, but now I crumpled into my seat. "Do...does...Jim...know?"

"Yes, the doctors are telling him now. I wanted you to know right away."

I did my best to hold back a sob. "What do I do now?"

"Get here. But, don't rush here. This process can take quite a while. But how about you start by calling Jim?" I could hear her smiling through the phone.

"Thank you. Just thank you. Thank you so much!"

"Drive safely, TJ. We'll see you later, okay?"

"Okay. Thank you. Thank you." I hung up and called Jim's cell.

It was a phone call where the feelings were louder than words. Jim was crying so hard he could barely breathe. He had been a rock throughout most of this his whole ordeal. Now, he had finally let go.

"I get to live I get to live I get to live." He sobbed, "They... j-j-j-just told me."

I nearly choked on my own tears. "I am so happy for you. Madeline told me. I am coming, baby. I am coming up now."

"Okay. Okay. Please come. Please come now."

I looked at my office phone. I saw Milly was still on hold. I clicked over. "Milly, I have to go."

"Is everything okay?"

I scrambled to put a full sentence together. "Yes — no — yes — liver. Liver for Jim."

"Go, okay. Just go!"

"Okay." I shut down my laptop and shoved it in my bag. I grabbed my purse, keys and a coat. I was hyperventilating as I ran down the hall to the VP who ran the office. "I have to go."

Harry took one look at my face and knew this was something big. "Oh my God. Is Jim okay?"

"It's liver. Jim's liver."

"Do you need a ride?"

"I've practiced for this. I can do it." I could barely form words anymore. I could barely think.

No matter how many times I had thought through this moment, I could never have predicted how getting *The Call* would feel. I felt foggy and elated. I had to get to my man, but I'd forgotten how to get to hospital.

Phone. Phone knows hospital. Make phone tell hospital.

Purse. Phone. Open map app. App map. Make find hospital. I can't type address. Fingers not going.

Where hospital?

My hands were shaking so badly I dropped the phone.

As I reached down and fumbled around on the floor of the driver's seat to find the phone, blood rushed to my head. I forced my mouth to say: "TJ. You are in shock. You need to breathe now."

Deep breath.

I made my mouth speak out loud again: "You cannot be in shock now. This behavior right now is self-indulgent and inefficient."

I felt my brain and mouth working together again. Things were coming back into focus. I was back online.

Liver. Hospital. Jim. What you'd planned for. You know what you're doing. Now execute.

City Hospital, Jim's Room

1:00 p.m.

When I arrived, Jim and I took one look at each other and both started crying all over again.

They had made a liver offer — which Jim had accepted.

A lot of things could happen, most of them bad for Jim, between the offer acceptance and the transplant surgery.

There is often a brief ceremony when a donor gives the gift of life. During the organ donation process, specially trained transplant teams treat the donor with care.

Th recovery team run recovered organs (as a donor may save more than one life) through a series of tests. This process helps to identify conditions that may have been unknown to the donor. The aim here is to transplant a healthy organ into a very ill individual. While the organ may be a match in every other way, undiscovered problems would disqualify it.

Recovery teams then package the organ for transport — yes, sometimes in coolers — and carried by hand by an organ recovery specialist. In Jim's case, the specialist would deliver it from the donor's hospital to City Hospital. Delays meant Jim's doctors would call off the transplant.

6 p.m.

The organ has arrived.

Jim's surgeons then did their last checks. They confirm the organ is in good shape. They also examine the physical characteristics to get a sense of any anatomical issues they might face to get the new organ to fit.

Through the long day, the transplanted team braced Jim and I for the possibility of disappointment. While Jim had a constellation of people all over the country working to make this happen for him, sometimes things don't happen as planned.

Nurses shared that many people make it as far as the operating room, only for doctors to call off the procedure. We both projected cool optimism while kept worries to ourselves.

We didn't share the news broadly yet because we didn't want to manage anyone else's feelings of disappointment if it didn't work out. Jim's feelings were the only ones that truly mattered. We needed to protect his heart.

But, with every minute that went by, we allowed ourselves to feel just a little more excited. We allowed hope in.

Because he had been all set for discharge and another liver patient needed his bed, the medical staff found Jim a bed in the trauma unit. A very amiable man with an eye aliment was Jim's new roommate.

Jim had the bed by the window and there was a steady stream of doctors and nurses coming in and out to see him.

One of the visitors who stopped by was the custodian for the liver ward. We had gotten friendly during our frequent visits and he asked if he could come in and pray for us. While we're not very religious, he clearly was, and we were deeply moved by his beautiful prayer.

Team Kidney came by to say hello.

Some of the nurses from the liver ward popped in to wish Jim good luck.

The time ticked by and the reports rolling in were good.

8 p.m.

A friendly but harried trauma nurse came in.

"I hear you're having some surgery tonight. We need to get you into a shower."

"You look pretty busy." I said, taking in her weak smile and the dark circles under her eyes.

"Bit of a crazy night."

"Would you mind if I help him?"

"That would be great. It would probably make him happier, too."

She stepped out to grab the necessaries.

"Jim, this may sound weird, but do you want me to take, um, a before picture."

"Of me looking so good?" He raised his eyebrows jokingly.

"I'm not sure if you'll want to remember this, but if you do want to, you'll have it."

"Okay. I'd show you my best side, but there really is no best side."

He slung his feet over the bed, and we took a picture — one that was just for him. One that showed how much he was about to overcome.

The nurse returned bearing an armload of towels and Dial soap. She then helped me get Jim into a wheelchair and directed us to the showers.

Despite all of his hospital stays, this was the first time Jim had ever been in a hospital shower. Frankly, I didn't know they had them.

It was a floor-to-ceiling tiled blue room with a shower stall large enough to hose down a racehorse.

Jim and I both made jokes that it was the perfect size to accommodate his ascites-accented girth.

Jim sat on the shower bench. (More like a shower couch. Seriously. The stall was huge.) I helped by handing him soap and washcloths. It was one of the coldest showers Jim had ever taken. It was definitely not a spa experience, but Jim was glad to be clean after lying in a hospital bed for days without a real wash up.

We were cracking a steady stream of jokes. Hope is a drug, and we were so totally high.

9:30 p.m.

Dr. Wilcox came into Jim's room all smiles.

"Well, I just checked out your new liver and it looks like we're a go."

"It's really happening?" Jim asked in a voice so soft and tentative you could barely hear it.

"Yes. You're getting a new liver tonight."

We cried. Again.

"Well, I'm off to home to take a hot bath."

"Wait. Are you serious?" I laughed, confused out of my mind.

"I need to be nimble for this. I will be back, though. You can count on it."

10 p.m.

An orderly came by, grabbed the edge of his bed, kicked off the breaks, and told Jim he was about to have the ride of his life.

As he deftly steered Jim's bed into elevators and through hallways, I walked alongside. Jim had a beaming smile for everyone and waved at passers by. This was his victory lap.

The surgical suite waiting room was dark when we arrived. It was after 10:15 p.m. The day surgeries were long gone. It was just Jim and me. It was one of those moments when silence is just fine. Hope doesn't always need words.

Finally, a member of the surgical team came to collect him. The nurse had her hair pulled into a surgical cap and was all smiles. It was showtime.

I looked Jim straight in the eye and said, "I love you. And, you've got this."

"I love you. And, I do." He winked.

Standing in the dark, I watched as the nurse wheeled Jim down a long, dazzlingly bright hallway.

It felt like goodbye and hello at the same time.

City Hospital, Lobby

I didn't wait around after that. The surgical team made me go home. I was no good to them if I couldn't wield a scalpel.

Those were the rules. Caregivers were to go directly home and go to bed. I could report back in seven or eight hours. They'd call if something went awry.

I wanted to follow the doctor's orders to the letter, but there was one more thing I had to do before I left.

I knew the hospital had a chapel. But, in truth, I was too bone weary to walk around and find it so late at night. Instead I consoled myself with the fact that the donor could very well have had a different belief set anyway. There was no guarantee he or she chose to frequent church. As I walked out the door at City Hospital, I walked up to a tree of life sculpture they had in the lobby, one which celebrated those who had given to the University. It reminded me of the design motif they used at the New Jersey Sharing Network and other organizations to celebrate those who had given the gift of life.

Not knowing what to do or how to start, I walked over to the wall, put my hand on it and thought of the person who made a choice to give and to live on in another.

I thought about that beautiful life.

I thought about the beautiful life their gift would allow us to have.

Just when I thought there weren't any more tears, I found some more.

Facebook Group
Jim's Liver Party
March 5

TJ: "*Please pardon any spelling mistakes. It's a little before 7 a.m. on Wednesday I'm dictating this into my phone as I drive back to the hospital. Want to give you that bit of behind-the-scenes. Yesterday, Tuesday, at 11 a.m. I received a call from the transplant coordinator. A liver was identified. After that, very, very many steps took place. We were told to hope for the best but be prepared for disappointment. I suppose that's why we erred on the side of caution with respect to letting folks know about this fantastic gift. Jim was wheeled into surgery at about half past 10 p.m.*

"*I've learned that all four of the transplant centers surgeons will be working on him. They are some of the best brains in the country. Also, given that they haven't done a transplant surgery in about a month, all of them were well rested an itching to cut.*

"The surgery itself lasts between seven and ten hours. This is followed by about two hours in the recovery room. Jim will then be moved to the Surgical Intensive Care Unit (SICU). It is there I will finally be able to see him. The surgery is pretty epic, so he will be unconscious for the next 12 to 36 hours depending on his condition so his body can meet its new friend.

The overall hospital stay should be between seven to ten days. After all the tubes come out (of which, I have been warned there are many), the doctors will be keen to get Jim on his feet. So, I expect the next few days will be about shuttling back and forth to the hospital."

This hospital stay is followed by a few weeks of at-home recovery. Following surgery, infection is a very serious concern. I am hoping my germophobic tendencies will finally be of some benefit. More to follow. Much love and thanks for your support. Today is a day of gratitude."

CHAPTER 13: MARCH 5

City Hospital, SICU Waiting Room

I knew from my years in the public relations field that sometimes not telling anyone much of anything is the best plan of action.

Wouldn't it be great to share the news when there was positive news to share?

We only told the immediate family about the surgery. In the morning, while I suspected his surgery was winding down, I let the small group of friends and relatives know who followed *Jim's Liver Party* on Facebook.

My plan was to arrive at the hospital at 7 a.m. In the best-case scenario, they would have concluded his transplant at 5:30 a.m. and they would let to see him at 7:30 a.m.

7:15 a.m.

I checked in with the nurse's station at the Surgical Intensive Care Unit (SICU — or as I, in my elated/exhausted state read it, "sick you").

The nurse called down to the operating room. Jim was still in there. Beyond that, there was no report.

She directed me to the SICU waiting room, a room in the hospital's basement with all the charm of...well, a hospital basement.

The waiting room was beige with a double ring of chairs that circled the room. Its only distinctive feature was a large, wall-mounted television set which looked as if it had seen better days. At this early hour, I was its only occupant, save the TV tuned to a flashy Spanish-language game show with the sound cranked all the way up.I looked around for a remote. Finding none, I felt around the TV to find a button or knob to turn down the volume. When I found the buttons, a metal strip covered them - same for the off button. The plug was also firmly bolted into the wall. I secretly wished a screwdriver-wielding thief would appear.

Not wanting to miss the news when it came, I found a seat directly across from the open door and settled in for the short wait.

9 a.m.

My parents had offered to wait with me, as did several friends, but I turned them down.

I am a pretty good worrier. I do it quietly. I'm not terribly theatrical about it. I am patient about the doctor's time. I don't pester for updates. If there was a career field and company associated with hospital waiting, I would be CEO. I didn't need a wing man for this.

Also, there wouldn't be much payoff for the visitor. They would spend a few hours of waiting with me and then the grand finale would be their seeing a (purposefully) unconscious Jim. I would rather they see him when he is awake.

Nah. This waiting stuff was official wife territory.

The doctors urged me to sleep, but I'd done little of that last night. I was just too wired, so today, I was running on about two hours of it. I asked my parents instead to head to my house. I realized I would be pretty wiped out and seeing them at the end of a long day would be nice.

No word on Jim, though.

10 a.m.

Still no word.

Noon

Nurse Madeline, transplant coordinator who called to give me the news yesterday, stopped by to say hi. She — thankfully — came bearing an update.

Dr. Wilcox shared with her that things were going well. The surgical team just needed a bit more time.

1 p.m.

Nada.

2 p.m.

Still in the Operating Room. Still no word.

The calls and texts started rolling in from *Jim's Liver Party* folks.

That he wasn't out of the Operating Room yet was cause for concern, but I wore a brave face and employed liberal use of *Jazz Hands!*

Most conversations went something like this.

Friend: What's that noise? Are you at a car show?

Me: I think it's, "Sabado Gigante?"

Friend: Jim likes Spanish shows?

Me: Not Jim. Waiting room. He's still in surgery.

Friend: Wasn't he supposed to be out this morning?

Me: Yeah, but you know how these things go, right?

Friend: Sure.

Me: He's doing great.

Friend: Do you want me to come up there and wait with you?

Me: No. I'm great, too. He will be out really soon.

3 p.m.

No update.

The phone rang.

"I've got a sitter," Reagan said. "I'm coming up."

"There's no need. He's great. I'm great —"

"No, you're not. I will see you in about an hour."

4 p.m.

Reagan arrived.

"Sit," She said, snapping into bossy mom mode once more.

"I am sitting."

She nodded. "Stay sitting. Eat this." She produced a plastic bag of granola bars and yogurt. That was the first moment I realized I hadn't eaten since yesterday morning. I devoured it like a ravenous wolf. "It was all I could find in my office fridge," she said apologetically. "What's up with Jim?"

"Nothing," I said through a mouthful of yogurt. "I've heard nothing."

The waiting room was now packed. Reagan made someone shift over a seat so she could sit next to me. "Want me to ask about his condition?"

"No!!!" I shouted, probably too loudly. I could just imagine Reagan giving her patented case of kick ass to a member of the hospital staff who then just happened to — oops! — give Jim slightly dented corneas instead of his new liver.

Instead, I called Madeline.

Facebook Group
Jim's Liver Party
March 5

TJ: "*Madeline (TC) connected with Dr Wilcox in the OR. He said they'd encountered some issues with bleeding, but that the situation was being managed and they are on top of it. (She encouraged me to not be alarmed. This is major surgery and these things happen.) They are still working on him. Dr. Wilcox will be out in an hour or so to talk to me..*"

City Hospital, SICU Waiting Room

Madeline shared that Jim had a connector problem.

Jim had severe ascites at the time of transplant. What this meant is the connectors between the new organ and Jim's veins and arteries didn't exactly match.

For illustrative purposes, think of what it would be like to connect a drinking straw (new liver) to a toilet paper roll (Jim's system). They *could* do it. They'd done it before. But this kind of thing could get tricky. Tricky takes time.

By this point, Jim had been in surgery for 16 hours.

5:30 p.m.

A family entered the waiting room earlier in the afternoon. They'd had an unfortunate circumstance. They — mom, dad, some adult children — had been out having lunch. I think it had been a family celebration of some kind.

At the meal, the youngest brother, age 24, suddenly got powerfully ill — the call-the-ambulance-and-take-him-to-the-nearest-hospital kind of ill. When he'd arrived, the doctors had taken him right into surgery to fix a malady only vaguely known to the family at this point.

I got the clear sense this wasn't their first choice of hospital. City Hospital has an outstanding facility and is staffed by exceptionally competent professionals, but it is generally known for trauma and (if you're in the special club, like us) liver transplants. I could safely guess that no one in that family had thought they would be spending their day here with their brother's life held in the balance. It was one of life's sudden and unpredictable awful events.

How someone reacts to their first experience with "life dealing you an unfair hand" tells a lot about their character. In traumatic times, people act out their worry, fear, and grief in different ways. I find that these tend to be magnification of someone's true nature. It was interesting to see this play out, in real time, with these siblings in the SICU waiting room.

There was action sibling. He would repeatedly step outside to work the phones and give others updates, saving his parents the trouble of telling the story of how things had gone wrong over and over again.

There was crying sibling. She would try to say something, which quickly devolved into inconsolable weeping for five minutes, after which she would raise her head say to no one in particular, "Why did this happen? Why?" in the same whispering voice the kid in *The Sixth Sense* says, "I see dead people." She'd then sprint out with the agility of an Olympian to find more tissues and then just as quickly resume her post and dab at her wet face.

There was questioning sibling. He repeatedly asked his parents and siblings about signs of disease trying to figure out what they and their brother had missed all along. He looked to be about 22 and could make a good doctor. Though, given his booming voice and exaggerated hand gestures, it was as if we all had been invited to the SICU community theater production of "House: The Musical."

Finally, there was self-involved sibling. It was clear she cared about her brother — a lot. But it was also clear she cared about herself quite a lot, too. You can always spot the self-involved because they are the ones who talked about time in a hospital.

"What time did they say they will they finish his surgery?"

"How long will it take him to get better?"

"How many more hours will this take?"

"I'd like to see him before I go. How much more of a wait before we can see him?"

At some point, she mentioned something about "the baby." I didn't see a baby, so I assumed she must be pregnant. "How long will it take the germs here to affect the baby?" she asked her barely holding-it-together mom.

Now take this running sibling commentary and make it last two straight hours. My nerves were frayed beyond repair. But at least it served as an excellent distraction from the Spanish game shows I had been listening to for over 10 hours at that point.

My biggest issue with this family was they were seat hogs. The elderly husband of an elderly patient having to stand because you are using two seats to put your coats and belongings on does not endear you to me.

I got up and gave the man my seat. Reagan gave me the "Why are you accommodating these assholes?" look, because best friends are life's truth tellers. Frankly, it was a good time for me to get up and stretch my legs, anyway.

Now that I had a partner in crime with me, I could safely walk and get a cup of go-juice without fear of missing a Jim update. I stopped to pee on the way to the cafeteria. In the ladies' room, the two sister siblings were chatting by the sink. I bypassed them and headed into the stall. The bathroom was the size of a postage stamp, so it was difficult to avoid overhearing them.

Self Involved Sister (SIS): "I just had to get away from that room. All of the germs, you know."

I got from the way she said "germs" that this was less about staphylococcus aureus and more a descriptor of her perceived quality of the waiting room's inhabitants, myself included.

Sob Sister (SS): "I'm just so worried about him. I just want to know why, you know? Why did this happen?"

I answered her in my head: Sister, I completely understand that. What I have learned from experience, however, is that those answers don't come easy, if at all. That T-shirt from the 1970s is true. Shit happens.

SIS: "Me too. I just don't know how much longer I should wait here. You know?"

SS: "I don't know how much longer this will t-t-t-take." I hear her grab some paper towels in lieu of tissues.

I flushed and came out to wash my hands.

"S-s-s-orry," SS sniffed. "I didn't notice anyone else in here."

"Do you work here?" SIS asked.

I looked around and realized she was talking to me. I gave myself a quick head-to-toe. Sloppy ponytail. Pair of loose black cotton pants. Well-worn sneakers. A V-neck H&M T-shirt and an unzipped pink polar fleece embroidered with one of my alma maters on the front. It didn't exactly say "hospital," but it didn't *not* say "hospital," either. I gave her the benefit of the doubt.

"No, I am a family member of a patient, but I have spent a good bit of time at the hospital. Perhaps I can help? What do you need?"

My money was on them asking where the cafeteria or chapel was, or maybe a question about parking, or where one of them could sneak a smoke. There's not exactly a visitor's guide for the hospital. I'd appreciated when people had helped me out in the past. Pay it forward, you know.

"I'm trying to figure if I should leave or not."

Now, she just asked another Jersey woman to give her opinion on something. She was about to unleash a dragon, so I made damn sure I got informed consent. "Are you asking my opinion on the matter?"

"Yes."

I appreciated that Sob Sister gave SIS some side-eye when she consented to my opinion on the matter. Did she often get her personal advice from random people in the bathroom? Whatever. She asked for it and I would give it to her.

"What's your primary concern?" I asked.

If she said, "My brother," I thought I might fall down dead with disbelief. But, of course, "Germs. I'm concerned about...the baby."

"Do you have a baby here?"

"No."

"Ah...then you must be pregnant. Congratulations!"

"I may be pregnant. I don't know. I'm just tired."

I saw she was wearing a wedding ring, so I guessed the pregnancy was planned. I wondered if she knew there are a wide range of products which let you pee on them to tell you if you are expecting. There are also blood tests for the impatient. I held off the nearly impossible impulse to give her a lesson in reproductive health. Instead, I got back to the matter at hand.

"I get that. Hospitals can be pretty exhausting. If you're concerned about germs, wash your hands thoroughly and frequently. There are also masks available. Just ask the SICU desk for one. If you want to be extra safe, take the clothes you're wearing now and throw them right in the hamper when you get home. Also, hop in the shower and wash your hair. I have one more question, though. What purpose do you serve by waiting here?"

"What?"

"Your original question was, 'Should I leave or not?' So, I'm asking you, 'How are you helping by being here?' I often find answering that question makes things clearer for me. I hope everything works out for your brother. I wish this hadn't happened to him or to all of you. But if you support each other, I know you'll all get through it. I've got to go get some coffee. Energy, you know? Take care."

As I was walking out, I heard:

"How did she know about our brother?"

"I don't know. M-m-maybe a psychic?"

"Or a total crazy."

When I returned, SIS had left and had taken her belongings — three chairs' worth — with her. I happily settled into one of the now-vacated seats.

At first, Reagan and I tried to keep up a string of chatter, but I couldn't anymore. Reagan then passed the time by posting updates on my behalf to *Jim's Liver Party*.

Finally, I saw Dr. Wilcox at the door. I had been here all day, and this was the first doctor who had showed up to the waiting room. Typically, a member of the SICU nursing staff would come and give waiting family updates or invite them to see their loved one.

"Hey, TJ, may I talk to you out here a minute?"

I stood up on wobbly legs. Reagan grabbed my arm.

"Do you want company?"

"No. This is something I need to do alone."

I followed him out the door and around the corner. I couldn't help but wonder if this was the bad news protocol. The walk was 15 steps but felt like 15 miles. Dr. Wilcox is a tall man. I looked up at his face, trying desperately to read it.

"It went great!" He said, breaking into a smile. "They're stitching him up now."

"He's alive?" I asked, not letting myself believe it.

"Yes, of course he is. And you can see him in about an hour."

My stomach did a somersault. "Did everything go okay?"

"There were some challenges. The fluid was a big one. We had to spend a few hours draining him of all that fluid. And then there were some bleeding issues. He's a strong guy, though."

"I heard the entire team was here. He got the all-star squad."

"It was our honor to make him healthy."

He directed me back to the SICU and told me someone would come get me shortly.

I'm not sure what happened — relief or exhaustion, maybe, but I walked back into the waiting room and cried in such loud boohoos I drowned out the sound of the TV. I felt the eyes of 30 people on me as I sat in my chair, curled into a ball, wailing in big, heaving, shirt-soaking sobs.

I heard whispers. I felt the guy in the seat next to me get up. Out of the corner of my eye, I saw a few others move away.

Reagan sat down next to me and put her hand on my back. She whispered in my ear. "Honey, is everything...okay?"

I didn't answer. I just sobbed louder.

"Is Jim...okay?" She said, a little more urgently.

My drunk-on-bliss brain could finally process that I was sending the exact opposite message of how I was actually feeling. I needed to find some words. Unable to lift my head yet, I mumbled into my lap, "He's fine. All okay." To emphasize, I gave her the thumbs up sign with one hand while wiping my face with the back of my other sleeve.

"Hey everybody! He's alive! He got the *transplant!*"

The room exploded into spontaneous applause.

SICU Patient Area, Jim's Room

If you've ever been in an ICU, the SICU was similar, just eerily quiet. Many patients were under sedation here, often having recently finished arduous surgeries.

The lights were low. You could hear the staff talking in urgent whispers.

Beds were in a large ring around a central nurses' station. There was a curtain between each bed and every occupant of those beds was hooked up to a variety of monitors.

I didn't immediately see Jim, but then a nurse pointed toward him.

Jim was in his own all-glass room, roughly the size of a one-car garage. You entered it through an alcove about one third the room's size.

Taking up most of the alcove was a set of computer monitors — roughly nine of them — on a rolling cart. The set-up was about the size of a basketball scoreboard. Seated behind the monitors was a nurse, lit by their glow in the dark room. If you've seen movies about NASA and space launches, you can get the general picture.

I stood back for a moment and watched her. She routinely checked each monitor one by one. When something caught her attention, she would stand up, head into Jim's room, and adjust one of the in-room machines.

I was slow to approach because I didn't want to throw her concentration. There seemed to be a rhythm to it. She had the look of an athlete at the top of her game. I just wasn't sure when it would be the right time to break in and ask if we could see Jim.

It is during times like these that Reagan's lack of personal boundaries comes in tremendously handy.

As I stared at Jim through the glass walls, Reagan's voice cut through the silence of the SICU. "Hi, I'm Reagan. This is my friend TJ. Is it okay for her to see her husband now?"

Where I expected scowling and snapping about maintaining concentration, we instead got a bright smile. "Certainly! I just need to walk you through a few procedures."

She advised us we couldn't stay long because Jim needed rest. That was true, I'm sure, but I also sensed it was her polite way of saying, "Please get the hell out in a reasonable timeframe so I can do my job and not kill your husband." That was all well with me. He was clearly in the hands of experts, and this team had a pretty stellar track record.

She told us he was heavily sedated. I quietly filed this under, "*No duh, I would hope so.*" Despite Jim's sedation, she encouraged us to talk to him, to let him know we were here.

She also said there were tubes and hook-ups all over the place and we should really avoid touching those. She warned me about a grizzly one on the right side of his neck. When you see people in the hospital, you're usually conditioned to see things on the arm or hand. Transplant patients apparently needed a more reliable hookup.

While she was giving us the rundown, Reagan and I donned hazmat outfits to match hers. That's not really what they were, but that's what they felt like. There were gowns to cover us from top to toe. There were gloves. There were shoe booties. The last touch was a pretty epic hospital mask which covered from the top of your nose to where your chin meets your neck. I got the sense these were a notch above standard issue.

We entered the room, and I took in the state of things. There were more monitors than I could reasonably count. Jim remained intubated, which obscured his mouth. Then I saw the other side of him. She was right to warn me. It looked as if he had a fuse box attached to his neck.

Jim looked as comfy as the situation would allow. The team did a good job with the covers and pillows, tucking him in nicely for a short winter's nap. Normally, I would fiddle with his covers. But there was nothing to fiddle with. And I didn't want to do any jostling of this.

I looked at him lying there. I thought about what he had been through. I thought about how many people were rooting for him and taking care of him. I considered all the steps he'd taken to come to this moment. There were so many thoughts, I found myself with nothing to say.

As if reading my mind, Reagan whispered, "You should say something."

"I don't know what to say!" I whispered back.

"Do you really want my voice to be the first voice he hears?"

I cleared my throat. I didn't need to. But isn't that how most poignant speeches started?

"Hi."

I could see Reagan rolling her eyes over her mask.

"I'm here and Reagan is here... and...and...you're great, honey. The doctor said you did great. I'm not sure if you can hear me but you're very brave and I'm really, really proud of you." I paused and the silence pressed in on me. "And you have a really big set of wires on the right side of your neck so please don't touch them."

Another Reagan eye roll followed this.

"They told me I can't stay long because you need to rest. There's this really nice nurse here who is sitting behind something out of Star Trek, and it's pretty stellar. I wish you could see it."

I took a deep breath.

"I know this has been a long road, but you need to rest now. Tomorrow, Mom, Dad and I are going to be here to see you, okay?"

I rested my hand on one of his calves, the only place I could find that wasn't attached to something.

"I love you. I love the shit out of you. And the cats say hi." I gave a quick wave with my other gloved hand, realizing belatedly he couldn't see it. "Okay, babe, we're going to go now."

I gestured to Reagan to see if she wanted to say anything.

"Hey, Jim!" Reagan broke in loudly. "You look real good! Okay. Bye for now!"

It was now my turn for the eye roll.

Reagan and I walked together to the front door of the hospital. It was close to 8:30 at night. Reagan had to rush out the door to go pick up her son. No one expected this day to be such a marathon, so I asked her to please thank her mother and sister for me. They'd covered the babysitting duties.

I paused in the lobby for a minute to text my parents I was coming home.

Facebook
TJ's Status Update
Jim's Status Update
March 5

TJ: "After a grueling 17-hour surgery, Jim has been successfully transplanted. Hallelujah!"

Our House, Kitchen

That night, I drove home with the windows open. It was frigid out, but I just needed to inhale some fresh air. I had been breathing in hospital air too long. I had been breathing in fear and anxiety and worry. I needed to fill my lungs and my heart and my very soul with something different.

This would normally be the time to turn on my tunes. But I needed something poetic, soothing and profound. I quickly realized not a single piece of music ever written could capture how I felt at this very moment. It was beautiful and complicated. If you ever had to explain to someone from another planet the very essence of the human experience, this was it.

I pulled in the driveway and saw my parents' familiar car.

I walked into the house, marched into the bedroom, threw my hospital clothes into the hamper, took a scalding hot shower and washed my hair. Then I tucked myself into the comfiest PJ's my drawer had to offer.

When I walked into the kitchen, Mom had put out a dinner of all of my favorites. Dad poured me a drink. When I gestured *just a little bit more* and pointed to the glass, he didn't hesitate. We are a family who never lets anyone drink alone, so there was a round for everyone.

As I ate the delicious home-cooked food, I told them about my day. I told them everything. Some of it was probably a repeat from our texts and calls throughout the day. But they never complained. They let me talk. As only parents can do, they listened with rapt attention and treated it as if it was the greatest story ever told.

Because for me, it was.

For Jim, he gets to start a whole new story. And that was damned good too.

I knew the work wasn't over. Recovery would not be a picnic. But, today?

Today, I would savor this victory.

For him. For us.

I raised my glass, "To Jim!"

Mom and Dad echoed, "To Jim!"

"And God bless us, every one," my mom added.

CHAPTER 14: MARCH 6-12

City Hospital, SICU, Jim's Room

Patients are told and retold that they will wake up in the hospital with a tube shoved down their throat. This is intended to come right out when the patient becomes conscious, but the first few moments may feel disorienting.

When Mom, Dad and I made the trip up at 9 a.m. the next morning, Jim was still asleep. When I said, "Good morning, Jim," he started moving around a bit, seemingly agitated.

"Well, he is starting to wake up and clearly has a lot to say to you. Let's get him more comfortable," the nurse said.

When I asked Jim later what was happening in his head he said it felt as if he was waking up from a really long, vivid dream. While he was semi lucid and waiting for the doctor to remove his breathing tube, he'd dreamed up a whole comedy thriller in his head about a charming rogue who was dating the daughter of a funeral director who was secretly disposing of bodies for the mob. Jim saw Seth Rogen in the lead. The crooked funeral director — think of a Ted Knight in Caddyshack type — hated Seth Rogen, and when Seth Rogen found out the funeral director was crooked, a hilarious cat-and-mouse chase ensued. Would the daughter side with her father or Seth Rogen? Would Seth Rogen escape after Ted Knight sealed him in a coffin as revenge? We'll never know, because Jim woke up before he could finish his mental screenplay. The nurses talked him through the process and kept him calm.

The nurses invited us in a few minutes later, fully dressed in our hazmat gear. Jim was hooked up to about 50% fewer things than last night. His color had mellowed from lime green to a pale yellow. The unfamiliar look was wonderful, if jarring. Jim had the look of a man who had just come from an all-night fraternity party — scruffy, smiley and in desperate search of pancakes.

Jim's transformation was remarkable considering, just a little over twelve hours ago, he had people's hands inside his abdomen rearranging his insides.

"Oh my God. Hi." I said, sounding like a giddy teenager.

"Good morning! It's morning, right?"

"Hello, Jim!" My mom chimed in.

"Hiya Mom and Dad. How do I look?"

"Normal, actually." My mom replied. "Does that sound weird?"

"A lot less yellow?" I added, smiling.

"You have been on one hell of an adventure. How do you feel?" Dad asked.

"Good. Really good."

I beamed. "Do you have any questions?"

"Not right now, but I will."

"So...wow. I don't even know where to start."

Jim laughed. "Well, right now is a new start, isn't it?"

We all smiled.

"Can I get you anything?"

"Is that Jell-O?"

"Looks like it."

"Is it for me?"

I turned to the nurse. "Is it for him?"

"It sure is."

While he was noshing his first meal post-transplant, we took a selfie. We used my head to block the enormous box still on the right side of his neck.

Facebook
TJ's Status Update
Jim's Status Update
March 6

TJ: "Sitting up and eating Jell-O. Huzzah!"

Facebook
TJ's Status Update
Jim's Status Update
March 7

TJ: *"Friday Update: Surgical ICU now trying to throw James Condon out because he's just too damned healthy. (Will have him in a regular unit no later than tomorrow.) I also just saw him hose an entire plate of lasagna. Considering how this week started, that was a sight to behold."*

Facebook Group
Jim's Liver Party
March 9

TJ: *"Sunday Update: Here is the latest medical and personal scoop: Jim is now out of SICU and in the regular liver ward. He has been on solid foods for two-plus days and everything seems to be in working order. He has a bit of fluid in his lungs, but given the length and complexity of his surgery, doctors told us to expect this. Jim is taking the exercise and rehabilitation thing very seriously. He is really busting his butt to work through the pain (of some pretty major abdominal surgery!) and complete the milestones which will move him along the road to recovery (e.g. breathing exercises, sitting upright, small steps). He is currently on insulin, as one of the anti-rejection drugs spikes his blood sugar. Again, doctors said to expect this. Special thanks to my parents (who arrived on the day of the surgery, departed today, and will return to assist me with discharge).: I'm trying to balance Jim's care with a part-time work schedule. So far, so good. But at this very moment? It's going on 7 p.m. and I think that is as swell a time as any to take advantage of the quiet and crawl into bed with hot tea and a book. Much love, Liver Party!"*

City Hospital, Liver Ward, Jim's Room

Those first few days were an excited blur.

From a surgical standpoint, Jim just kept beating every recovery milestone.

Optimism was the order of the day, which was a delightful treat after so many months of dread and worry.

Jim, meanwhile, was handling the recovery stuff with marked enthusiasm. We all wanted Jim to come home the healthiest version he could be of someone who just got brand new guts.

Pneumonia was the big watchword now. Jim became instantly chummy with his respiratory therapists. Any "inhale this," or "blow that," and Jim was on it.

As the caregiver, it left me to handle, well, just about everything else.

Jim's move into the "normal guy sick room" felt like graduation, but also the moment shit was about to get real from a caregiver perspective.

Gone was the 24-hour team. Now Jim and I were much more on our own. SICU was the toddler bike. The regular ward was the regular bike with training wheels. As the day of his discharge loomed, I feared the moment those wheels were ripped right off.

On Tuesday, I spent all day in the hospital with Jim, meeting with doctors and nurses about his ongoing care. Getting someone to transplant is a lot different from helping someone recover from a transplant. Each offers different challenges and calls on a new skill set. I needed to adapt. Quickly.

This entire process reminded me of college exams — where you had to cram and cram and cram so you could nail one exam, only to purge that knowledge so you could stuff your brain with fresh information and rock the exam for your other class. One of the distinct advantages of going to a liberal arts college was that you learned how to become temporarily smart in Astronomy, Theater, History and German in a compressed time period. It was a gift which came in handy now.

I was tired and still had a mountain to climb. I had been at the hospital every day, for nearly full days, for seven days straight.

I was advised that Jim would be discharged later that week — Thursday, most likely.

My plan was to skip the hospital on Wednesday, head into the office for a few hours in the early morning to close things out and then devote the entire day to home readiness. His room was in fine shape and the house in good order, but I still had a lot of last-minute things to do. The short list included:

Pet Re-accommodation: I needed to get the cats settled in their basement apartment. This would require cajoling and treats.

Germaphobe's Paradise: I had stocked up on the mountain of supplies I would need to keep the environment at home as germ-free as possible—furnace filters, humidifiers, gloves, masks, disinfecting wipes, garbage bags, etc., etc., etc. I needed to strategically place these items all around the house.

Medical Supplies: Jim's incision was no joke. Picture something enormous and oozy. I had a full complement of gauze and medical tape to keep him from popping open *Total Recall* Kuato-style.

The *And Now for Something Completely Different* Diet: The transplant surgery had apparently pissed off Jim's kidneys. A lot. We needed to soothe them by feeding them stuff they enjoyed. The problem was that the diet (minus the salt restrictions that Jim was already accustomed to) represented a 180-degree nutritional shift. Stuff like potatoes, avocados, bananas, oranges, spinach, cantaloupe, beans, broccoli, tomatoes and most whole grain things were suddenly evil, as were dairy in all forms and dark-colored soda.

On the Road Home from City Hospital

When I was driving home on Tuesday, I got an unexpected call from the hospital.

"Hello."

A person I'd never met before from the hospital went straight to business, "I'm calling about your medication training and pickup."

"Oh, okay. Jim's discharge is on Thursday afternoon. How about Thursday morning?"

"Thursday, you say? Well then, it will have to be tomorrow."

"But, I didn't plan to be there tomorrow..."

"Are you saying you won't prepare for your patient's discharge? The person in your care?"

"Wait? What?"

"Yes, and you need to prepare."

My voice went steely, "I assure you I am quite prepared."

"You are not if you don't understand how to administer his medication. You need to be here tomorrow. At noon."

"But I was just up there. Just a few minutes ago. Can I turn around and come back?"

"The staff can't see you now."

"But I have things to do tomorrow."

"This is your responsibility. We will see you tomorrow. At noon." She hung up.

Now to say that I was pissed off did not begin to categorize the surge of fury I experienced.

It was the questioning of the commitment that got me. It was the suggestion that by working or by taking time away from the hospital *to get someone ready to come home from the hospital* was reason for disappointment.

I spent the next several hours in a simmering rage. At the supermarket, I threw boxes in the cart. I angry-cleaned my house while listening to *Nine Inch Nails*. In the early morning, I growled at my coworkers. I seethed during my entire ride there and all but stomped into Jim's hospital room, our appointed meeting place.

City Hospital, Jim's Room

Jim wasn't in his room. It was just me, a nurse whom I'd never met before and a pharmacist who fell into the same category. I had zero idea if either of the people before me was the lady from the hospital who'd called me, but my fury just didn't care.

"I've left work. I've stopped preparing the house for Jim's arrival home. I am here as you instructed. During the middle of the day. Now, how may I be of help to you?" My voice was so icy I'm surprised snow didn't start falling. Then they had to go and be really nice to me.

"Hi, it's nice to meet you," the pharmacist said.

"Same here," the nurse added. "We really appreciate you coming in today."

"We know you're really capable, but this stuff isn't easy. We just wanted to make sure you had help to understand it all."

"And this is the first time we were both available at the same time!"

"Because he's doing so well, he's going home sooner than we thought."

This was the moment when I felt like a complete and utter tool. I saw their lunch bags on the little table in the corner and realized this was a meeting crammed into an already long day for them. This may even have been their lunch hour that they were giving up for Jim, and for me.

"I'm really sorry. I lost my head a moment. You're doing your jobs and I was a little...frosty."

"It's all good. We know you're very committed to his care," the nurse assured me.

"That's why you're here," the pharmacist said.

"Okay, then. School me on the drugs!"

Thank. Jesus. I. Took. The. Ride. Here.

I'd brought a notebook with me. I travel with one all the time. But, I took so many notes I filled remaining five pages and had to write on the back cover of the book to capture them all.

Jim would be on 18 different medicines for the next month, all administered in different ways and at different times of the day, on a very strict 24-hour schedule.

There would be pills (natch), liquids for swallowing, liquids for swishing and spitting, ointments for smearing, and possibly things to inject.

I would also have to take him in for blood tests two times a week. The liver center would call me with instructions if things needed fine-tuning. If I didn't hear from them, I was to call them to confirm I should continue to stay the course.

They told me in the nicest, most positive and encouraging way that if I gave Jim the wrong stuff at the wrong time, I would kill him.

"Do you have any questions?" the nurse asked.

I felt as if I had just sat through a twelve-hour exam. I was certain if I dabbed my ears, I would feel grey matter leaking out. I had many questions—about a thousand—but I didn't even know where to begin. "Not at the moment. You were most thorough. I just need to take all this in."

"Totally understandable," the pharmacist said. "When you have questions, we're here for you."

"Thanks again for making the trip."

"If you wanted to do the pickup now, the hospital pharmacy will be ready for you."

They grabbed their lunch bags and departed. I had completely lost my appetite. Just moments after they left, a nurse wheeled Jim back in.

"This is a surprise!" He said, cheerily. "I didn't expect to see you today."

"Just had to come in for some...training." My heart was beating a mile a minute.

"Feel like watching me get a breathing treatment?"

"Um...not right now. Hey, did you know you're going to be on a lot of drugs?"

"I know. Anti-rejection drugs. Rest of my life."

"But, now. Like, when you come home."

"I figured a few."

"A lot."

"You're all good with that, right?"

"So. Very. Totally."

So. Totally. Not.

"Honey, I gotta go. They told me to go to the hospital pharmacy to get your drugs."

"Wait, you won't hang around? Even for lunch?" He seemed disappointed, but my breathing had gotten shallow. I needed to get out of there before full on panic set in.

"Nah. I gotta get the house in shape for your triumphant return!"

City Hospital, Pharmacy

The nurse and pharmacist had given me directions to an onsite hospital pharmacy. One doesn't notice a pharmacy at a hospital. I never gave much thought to where the drugs actually came from. Drugs at a hospital always just showed up, like Santa and his elves leaving presents under the Christmas tree in the middle of the night.

It turns out it was a nondescript building I had passed several times before but never noticed. The building had clearly seen better days, and then even better days before those better days.

This wasn't a *let's browse for greeting cards* kind of pharmacy. This was a *get your meds and get out* kind of pharmacy. Pharmacists worked in a large, windowed booth. They set this booth about two feet above the floor, so it had this quality of the pharmacists looking down on the visitors — either benevolent drug angels or judgmental overlords, depending upon what sort of mood you were in. *Wait, is that bulletproof glass?*

There were a scant few products outside of the windowed booth, mostly just cough drops and other kinds of cough drops. All of the stuff with any true medicinal value was kept behind the window. It gave the place an air of desperation — the kind of place where someone would swipe Tylenol. The hospital is in an urban center that is home to law offices, an airport and a bunch of people barely scraping by. I waited while a lady argued about her $2 prescription. I couldn't tell if she'd paid for it and was unhappy or wanted it and was short the $2. All I knew was the confusion escalated as fast as the yelling.

I wanted to go home and decided a two-dollar investment might bring her joy and help me reclaim some time. I reached for my wallet.

A man in line stopped me, "I see what you're doing. I wouldn't do that."

I looked at him quizzically.

"Don't pay for her prescription. That's Crazy Alice. She just likes to yell."

"Got it. Thanks for the tip."

He was one of two other customers in line in front of me. They both looked as if they needed a blanket and some human kindness. They were just stretched thin and tired. I assumed this was one of the last stops on their already long day. By that point I had nothing left in the human kindness department, but I wanted to muster some. They took the first customer in line and then my new friend stepped up to the counter. I listened to hear what he owed and again reached for my wallet. Perhaps I could make this guy's day a little easier. The pharmacist clearly recognized him, however, and handed him a bag with a smile, not asking for cash. "See you in a few days," the pharmacist said as he headed out the door. I hoped those next few days were happy and healthy ones for him.

Now it was my turn. I stepped up to the counter. The pharmacist appeared surprisingly chipper for a man who had just done a round with Crazy Alice.

"Just you today?" He asked after I gave him my information.

"Yep," I said, looking around the empty pharmacy. "Just me."

"I meant to help carry things."

"I'm pretty burly. I think I can handle it."

"I'll bet you can. But this may take a few trips."

A few trips?

The first thing he handed me was a scale.

"I didn't order a scale. Is this my...um, stuff?"

The pharmacist responded brightly, "It's just a gift from us. You know, for the patient. The patient..." He looked at a nearby slip of paper, "James. James, right?"

"Then, thank you. From...Jaammes." His formal name felt weird on my tongue.

He then handed me a cheerful-looking box with butterflies on it and another the size of a loaf of bread, filled with needles.

"They told you to have sugar around, right?"

"Pardon?"

"Sugar. In case you give him too much."

It was then I remembered the lesson on Insulin. Some patients need it as they get used to their new liver. I took notes on it. But I had conveniently filed this knowledge under "*Nice to know, but won't need.*" I had clearly misfiled.

My mind then started going to that scene in *Pulp Fiction* where John Travolta has to jam Uma Thurman's character in the chest with a needle and it just sort of sticks out, hanging there. I then remember it wasn't Insulin. Epinephrine, maybe? Wait, is he getting some of that too? Must I administer the the Pulp Fiction treatment?

"Do you need any candy?"

"I think we're okay on sugar."

I vaguely remembered some rock candy we had lying around from when Jim was still eating. I figured it was dissolvable. I would have gone with orange juice ala *Steel Magnolias*, but now that was on the no-eat list.

The pharmacist then leaned down over the edge of the counter and handed over a bright red canvas bag. The bag was the size that would make a flight attendant look at you askance if you billed it as your carry on. I took it from him and smiled.

"Free bag, too? For Jaammes." It still felt weird to say.

"Yup. Free bag!"

This was the same pharmacy which had just argued with Crazy Alice about a nickel for a good fifteen minutes. I was glad she was not here to see this.

As this was going on, other people entered the pharmacy and queue up behind me in line. I heard a waiting woman whisper, "Oh dear! What on earth is that woman sick with?" and realized she was talking about me.

Keen to move things along, I handed him my credit card, the one which got me all those swell Amazon points. He took it and then said, "Let me go to the back for the rest."

The rest!?!

He merged about two minutes later with what I guess were the cold things, one of which looked like a two-liter bottle of soda.

"Well, this must be the mouthwash, then." I said, authoritatively. This was the only thing I actually remembered from the training.

He handed over the bottle with another smile. This man was either the most assertively cheerful person I'd ever met or totally high.

"Three times a day on this one. And keep it refrigerated. Do you live close to here?"

"I...wait, what?"

"Where do you live?"

Is this what a pharmacist flirting sounds like? No clue. I went full honesty on this one.

"Central Jersey."

"Is that far?"

"About an hour."

"Okay. Let me get you an ice pack, then."

Well, this was a love that could not be. He made his way to the register. "Okay! That will be $1,346."

Now, I knew this was coming. Though the lady who thought I was sick now probably thought I was dying. Crazy Alice would totally be losing her shit right now. I handed over my card.

Later, when I looked at the reconciled bill, I saw they just handed me the (pre-insurance) equivalent of $8,000 worth of medications. It was opportune, then, that the pharmacist used this moment to hand me one of those colorful Morning/Noon/Evening/Night pill boxes the size of a Buick.

"For James, too," he smiled.

"Thank you very much."

As I walked to the car, trying to see around my tower of pharmaceutical bounty, I kept saying one thing over and over again—part prayer, part mantra.

"Must not kill Jim. Must not kill Jim. Must not kill Jim."

Facebook Group
Jim's Liver Party
March 12

TJ: "Pardon any bad spelling. Dictating this into my phone. Just had my medication overview (for the next three months, he will be on 18 of them) and discharge training the hospital. All signs point to Jim being discharged tomorrow. I have asked my parents to come up and assist. We are also working to bring in a home nurse for care. Expect that may take a day or two to ramp up. *The most important thing is this: in order for liver patients to accept organ, their immune system must be suppressed. What this means is Jim is very, very, very susceptible to illness. We are taking every step to keep germs out of the house. Please do not visit if you are ill or have been around others who are ill. In the event you do stop over, please wash hands. And if you plan on touching Jim (meow!), glove up. Headed home now to finish room crap, laundry and as many other necessaries as I can before Jim's triumphant return. Much love to my liver party."*

CHAPTER 15: THE REST OF MARCH

Our House, Discharge Day

I knew Discharge Day was starting to go off the rails when it took over an hour just to get Jim into the house.

Dad was my co-pilot, as Mom was currently home battling a contagious aliment of her own. Since Jim was *Boy in the Bubble* for the next few weeks, anyone in close contact with Jim would need to have a clean bill of health and still be prepared to mask-up/glove-up when they were in close contact.

We pulled into the driveway at 4 p.m., the discharge process and subsequent drive home having taken the better part of five hours.

It was now Jim's big moment. Dad inched the car up the driveway so the back seat of the car opened out onto the paved walkway to the front door. I stepped out of the passenger seat, opened Jim's door, grasped his elbows (as the nurse showed me how to do) and counterbalanced him to a standing height.

Jim immediately grabbed his abdomen, presumably to double check his guts were not falling out. Once assured his insides were still inside, he took a step. When he tried to take another, he asked if he could rest a minute first. We stood there, arms linked in the cold, Jim huffing and puffing for about two minutes.

It would be another 59 steps, two stairs, and a little over an hour before Jim got to his room.

During this time, my dad got the car unpacked, started a load of laundry and called my mother. Then, before he could pour himself (and me) a well-deserved shot of bourbon, I dispatched him to the local pharmacy for Jim's pain pills and a few additional supplies.

The plan was to get Jim settled in bed, feed him dinner, and wake him when necessary for pills. What I didn't consider was the complexity.

Jim left the hospital with fluid in his lungs. Now imagine trying to cough this up with belly-wide surgical incisions. While he did need to move around and "exercise," even small things were a big deal to Jim. (Case in point: While he sat on the bed, it took both of us around 20 minutes to wrestle him out of his coat.)

There was also a problem with his drugs. A piece of advice I received was to get the first order of anti-rejection and anti-infection drugs from the hospital pharmacy but fill the pain pills closer to home. The latter may need to be refilled with greater frequency, and if Jim was in urgent need, I didn't want him to wait while I made the 2+ hour round-trip drive up north to get them.

The problem was, my local pharmacy did not have the pills—at least not in the specific dosage the hospital required. Thankfully, a few calls from the pharmacy to Jim's doctors and to the hospital gave them what they needed to adjust the prescription. The diligent pharmacist working Jim's case even kept the store open an extra half an hour so he could see this through for us.

Our House, Discharge Day +1

To start, we needed a routine. Here is how it went for Day 1 and the roughly 30 days that followed:

6:00 a.m.

I wake up to my alarm, shower and put on clothing of the elegant-sweatpants variety. I shovel a granola bar or other one-handed breakfast treat into my mouth. I head down to the basement to check on the cats and administer much petting.

6:45 a.m.

I don mask and gloves and then wake up Jim. I check his blood pressure and temperature. I clean off the mouthpiece of the breathing measurement device and hand it to him so he can puff into the pipe. I then hand Jim the lancet and glucose test strips so he can do a blood sugar check. The blood sugar testing machine then invariably reads the sample as insufficient and I go at Jim like a hungry vampire. I record all this information in a composition book on his bedside table. While I am doing this, Jim gets on the scale. I then record his weight. Jim resettles on the bed and I hand him a bottle of water and a pack of pills, his first set of meds for the day.

7:15 a.m.

I head to the kitchen to make Jim a cup of tea, some white toast (because kidneys!), and a diet-approved fruit and/or egg. I make myself a cup of coffee the size of a goldfish bowl.

7:30 a.m.

I bring Jim his breakfast. He eats while I do a quick wound check (yay, no oozing!) and the morning cleanup which involves a medical waste collection, a general waste collection, and a generous Clorox wipe of anything Jim or I have touched.

Once he's cleaned his plate (because nutrients!), I toss it in the garbage. We have become a nearly 100% paper plate I have given myself the gift of dishwasher avoidance.

8:00 a.m.

It's time for The Pillstravaganza! This 8:00 a.m. dose is focused on better breathing, fighting infection, and supplements. Highlights include Prednisone, Valcyte Calcium with Vitamin D, Magnesium Oxide, Vitamin C, and Vitamin E. There is also Docusate to counteract the so-totally awesome impact of Morphine on the digestive system.

On doctor-visit days, these pills are followed by teeth brushing and face washing, a shower for Jim, and a mad dash around the house for me to help get him ready.

On non-doctor-visit days, Jim takes his morning nap and I use the time to answer any truly urgent work emails and do the usual stuff that needs doing around the house. For most of his life, Jim has been a "sleep in weird positions" guy. He generally prefers to sleep with his face buried in a pillow, with arms and legs at all different angles while buried under a pile of cats. His current situation of sleeping sitting up at a 45-degree angle, uninterrupted, in a quiet room, to the soothing sounds of the ocean was slow torture. Still, this morning nap was essential to having him heal and also to avoid crankiness.

10:00 a.m.

This is the first dose of the day for the anti-rejection medications — Prograf and Cellcept. This is also the start of a new lifelong routine. For the rest of his life, at 10 a.m. and 10 p.m., Jim will need to take pills. As a post-surgical patient, the doses are big, variable and complicated. Frequent calls from the liver center have instructed me how much I should step up or back off the doses.

In these early, just-following-transplant days, Jim might take a quarter-cup full of pills for a single dose.

After pills, it is time for physical therapy. Jim has to get up and walk around staving off the pneumonia. We have a very modest-sized, ranch-style house and Jim tracks his progress by the room he can reach without too many huffs and puffs. A walk from the guest bedroom (his current residence) to the living room and back again is big doings.

This is usually also around the time of day we give him pain pills. Pain pills are very specifically not on the formal schedule because Jim takes them when needed. While Jim never abused them, if the pill said take every four to six hours, we were opening that bottle at three hours and 59 minutes. The pain was manageable, but intense.

Being sick takes so much from you, so little victories become very important. We were lucky enough to get this good piece of advice from one of the transplant coordinators: If you're doing the same or a little better than yesterday, you're doing phenomenally well. The goal is not dramatic improvements; the goal is steady progress. This can feel maddening to high achievers, but it's a much better measurement of success than benchmarking against other patients. If Jim could stand on his feet two more minutes than the day previous, that was progress, and each time I would shoot pretend confetti and streamers at him.

Exercise exhausted Jim, so when he finished, so we would get him settled in the living room. My dad and I had moved the recliner in there from the den so Jim could sit comfortably while also watching the big TV.

Jim would have preferred to sit there with a cat on his lap, but even I still had to glove up every time I touched him. Our cats are pretty chill, but I didn't think they would take to the mask and glove thing. Would it go over or under the whiskers?

After getting him settled, I go to the kitchen and figure out something for lunch. Maybe no-salt chicken soup? Maybe some no-salt peanut butter and jelly on cheap white bread (because whole grains were a no-no)? Maybe some fruit ice pops with steamed vegetables on the side?

I bring out the food to him while he relaxes in his recliner. He eats and then watches something with one eye while reading the news on his phone with the other.

2 p.m.

This was the time for even more pills, including a really annoying swish-and-spit drug which prevented thrush. You may be familiar with thrush as a mouth infection babies and the elderly get. Well, so do transplant patients! The drug had to be kept cold. I would give it to Jim in a paper Dixie cup, and he would do the best he could to spit it accurately into whatever receptacle I provided for him. I felt like a valet on *Downton Abbey*.

This was also the time for Jim's spa treatment (a.k.a. shower). Thanks to the power of Amazon, we now had a hospital bench in the shower, so Jim could clean up in relative comfort. Before getting in there, I'd remove the layers of medical tape and gauze and arranged the shower so that shower supplies, like antibacterial soap, were all within easy reach.

While he was in the shower, I'd set up a wound-maintenance station. After working together to get him out of the shower and dry, on went the new layer of bandages. Jim would hold the gauze with his free hand, while I worked the medical tape with my gloved fingers, swearing the entire time.

Usually, right in the middle of this, I would get a call from the liver center—typically from Elvia, the nurse who worked with Jim. Elvia was of Filipino descent. She loved God, her family, her patients and cute shoes, in that order. What she did *not* love was having her time wasted. I would scramble to find the notepad of Jim's vitals and a pen while she called out changes.

"New prescription. For the kidneys. Fludrocortisone. Every other day. Did you get that?"

"Every other day." I repeated.

"Give me his weight."

I did, and shared a bunch of other stats too.

"Okay. We are going to give him diuretics now." I scribbled furiously. "You'll get another prescription, too. But we need to watch his weight on this. Are you taking his weight every day?"

"Yes, ma'am." Elvia was like a tiny, benevolent drill sergeant. I would call her sir if she wouldn't find it weird.

"It's called Lasix."

I vaguely remember this from his previous hospital visit. "Isn't that what they give racehorses to, like, pee?"

"Yes."

"Yes?"

"Jim will pee like a racehorse."

"Got it."

"So, about the Prograf—"

"Hi, Elvia!" Jim called out.

"What was that?"

"Jim says, 'Hi.'"

A smile came into her voice now. She adored her patients, but Jim especially. "Tell him I hope he is feeling better. Talk tomorrow."

After this, I would run to the closet and pull out clothes for Jim so he could pick his preferences. Jim favors dark neutrals, but he was particular about them.

"Which one?" I asked, holding up two identical pairs of sweatpants.

"The blue ones would be great."

"Which blue ones?" I genuinely could not tell the difference.

"The ones you're holding in your right hand."

We would then get him dressed and resettled in the living room.

Conservatively, this bath, bandage, dress routine took about an hour-and-45-minutes, after which Jim would be pretty knocked out. Back to the chair he would go, so I could shift my attention to chores.

3:30 p.m.

This was my time for daily chores. Tasks would typically include a mix of the following:

Humidifier Cleaning: I had two heated-mist humidifiers which I ran constantly in the rooms where Jim spent the most time. The intent was to keep down airborne germs. The upside was they made the room a warm, skincare paradise. The downside was they required daily cleaning.

Trash Removal: Between gloves, masks and packaging detritus, we made a lot of garbage. To keep germs at bay, I was constantly running bags to the trash.

Dishes: Even with my firm commitment to paper-based dining, I somehow used more dishes than ever. I think it was because I would make myself a coffee, take it into whatever room I was in, take two sips and then forget about it, only to make another cup five minutes later.

Laundry: Towels were a one-time-use thing with Jim. I washed his bathrobes frequently. I also washed and changed his sheets every tother day. There were also the sheets and blankets that covered the furniture on which he sat. Even with well-tended bandages, sutures got a little leaky now and again. And there were the usual spills associated with sedentary living—the errant coffee slosh here, the sprinkle of crumbs there. It could get really yucky, really fast. My new commitment to cleanliness was a 180-degree turn for the woman who used to eat crackers in bed and washed her sheets once a semester in college.

Toilet and Shower Cleaning: Bathrooms are a germ factory. The bathrooms would get a daily scrub and spray down with disinfectant.

Pharmacy Management: This was when I would manage Jim's pill sorting and refills. I used the dining room table as my medical office. I devoted one side of the table to bills and the other side to pills. Every afternoon, I would glove up, mask up and get Jim's pills ready for the following day. What seemed to work best was a mix of labeled snack-sized bags and sandwich-sized bags. I would write the time of day on them with permanent marker. I would also write if something was in another part of the house. The bag would read something like: "10 a.m. + Fridge." Once these were in order by time of day, I would then do my refill check and call it in to the pharmacy.

After the first prescription fill at the hospital, I could stick with them or move the prescriptions to our local pharmacy. We had gone to our local pharmacy for years and I had really hoped to continue working with them, especially considering their heroic efforts during Jim's first day home. But Jim's prescriptions weren't run-of-the-mill stuff. Nevertheless, they took to the challenge of Jim's epic drug regimen with professionalism and gusto. The key was surprise avoidance. If we both stayed on top of it, I could stick with them and not have to take long trips up north. For the first few weeks, I talked to my pharmacy every day.

Online Medical Shopping: This is also when I would pick up other things we needed. Clicking around on Amazon yielded me a transport wheelchair that would get Jim from car to doctor's office door in record time. Even better? The chair was cheaper than a nice dinner out. I thought it was a sound investment, and it was at my door in under 48 hours.

5:30 p.m.

Dinner time. I tried to get Jim's dinner on the recliner-side-table before 6 p.m., because at 6 p.m. he would have to take oral medicine, which tasted awful. This is when I would recheck the list of what he could have, scan the pantry and figure out what the heck to put on the plate. Salt-free corn chips with a side of corn and red pepper salsa? Noodles with unsalted butter? With carrots on the side? I pulled out a paper plate, put his food on it and placed a folded a napkin on the side for impromptu elegance.

6 p.m.

Swish and spit time!

7:00 p.m.

Around this time, I would beg off of Jim's company and head to the kitchen. This is when the cats would have their upstairs time. I would open the basement door and they would run upstairs to meet me. I would feed them a cornucopia of canned delights and would feed myself whatever I could find. If I was lucky, I would find a Mom-made frozen meal. If I wasn't, dinner would be peanut butter smeared on stale crackers. I would eat my dinner seated in the remaining recliner in the den (part of the cat demilitarized zone) and both of the cats would pile on top of me. They were pretty starved for attention by this point and wanted time with their people. In between bites, I would pet them and tell them this situation wasn't forever. When they whined, I would play Da Bird with them until they were satiated, and I was ready to keel over.

8:00 p.m.

More supplements! And stool softeners!

I would like to say this was our couple time — the time for me and Jim to talk about our hopes and dreams for the future. But it was more like logistics planning while I took Jim's arm and he made his nightly stroll around the first floor. (We really had to keep those lungs happy.) Jim, never one to bottle up his thoughts, would use this time to tell me how he felt about everything — the relative comfort of the bed, the discomfort of the stitches. I would listen as attentively as one can at the end of a long day.

8:45 p.m.

After I got Jim settled, I would spend the next 45 minutes to an hour responding to work items. If a matter was pressing, I would set the alarm for 3 a.m. to tackle it in a few hours, because I always think best in the morning.

9:40 p.m.

Night-night time. I help get him ready for bed and tuck him in with everything he needs for sleeping, to be completed by no later than 9:59 p.m. Teeth. Jammies. Water by the bedside. Plugged-in phone. TV remote within reach. I think bedtime was Jim's greatest disappointment, second to my culinary skills. He is a *go-to-bed-at-midnight* guy. To him, anything earlier feels as if he is wasting the day. I am a *go-to-bed-at-8:30 p.m.* girl. This was my way of splitting the difference. It was also helping him get a full eight hours of rest. Well, this was part of how I justified it, because it was mostly true. The fact also remained that by 10 p.m., I was so tired I could barely form words anymore.

10:00 p.m.

I hand Jim his sack full of nighttime anti-rejection drugs. He tosses them back, washes them down with a bottle of water, and watches TV in bed.

10:01 p.m.

I'm sound asleep in my bed across the hall.

Our House, Home Office

I had four truly mandatory business trips a year. We were a small public company and the team who helped to file and report the earnings was smaller still. Four times a year, it became an *all-hands-on deck* situation.

My coworkers were incredibly sympathetic to my situation, but I think most quietly hoped Jim had the power to plan his illness around the Security and Exchange Commission's mandatory reporting cycle.

I needed to travel in the middle of April—in roughly four weeks. It was something of constant concern, because recovery is something which can't be forced or hurried. Recovery does its own thing. My plan was to be there with him every step of the way, but there would be a time in the future when I couldn't. This worried me more than a little.

One of the potential options was a visiting nurse.

Health insurance wouldn't cover the cost. They seemed to think every caregiver had the skills of a practical nurse coupled with unlimited time availability and a complete absence of personal needs such as sleeping.

The first days after abdominal surgery required round-the-clock help because there was a real chance Jim could get stuck somewhere. Let's say he was to sit in a chair, which was just a little too deep, and he needed to get up to go to the bathroom. Because his guts had been rearranged, and his abdominal muscles couldn't be counted on, Jim couldn't scooch. Jim could only grab and pull himself up, while keeping his chest perfectly straight and having his thigh muscles do the work.

Jim's blood pressure was also still a bit wonky, so getting up from any lying or seated position made him dizzy. Jim going "Timber!" was a real possibility I needed to guard against.

The point being: Solo time for Jim just wasn't in the cards right now. I started making calls. My first was to a nursing company whose name you would recognize from their frequent TV advertisements. The conversation went a little something like this:

"We'd love to provide care for Jim. Let me walk you through our services. [Insert prepared speech with liberal use of the word *compassion*.]"

"That sounds great. He'll need medication several times a day."

"Oh, our nurses don't administer medication."

"What happens if he needs to take medication?"

"They could get him the pill bottle and he would give himself the medication."

"Let's just say for discussion that he's a little loopy. Would they be able to read a chart I have of medication names and times and make sure he's taking the right thing?"

"That would be the patient's responsibility."

"I see. He also has some incision wounds that are healing. He needs the dressings changed twice a day."

"Our nurses don't do wound care..."

"Are you saying that's the patient's responsibility, too?"

"You got it! They would, as an example, hand him the gauze and tape and he could do it himself."

My next question was going to be...

"So, if he is having a heart attack and is too busy clutching his chest to go get the phone, would your team call 911 or would you hand him the phone so he could dial himself?"

But I had pity on the nice lady.

"Can your team members help him so he can get up and go to the bathroom or shower?"

"Absolutely. They just can't offer help washing or assist him in the bathroom."

"Okay. Self-wiping. Got it. Thank you."

After calling three other companies, I learned that this was just the way of things.

Yes, there were options available for more skilled nursing care — nurses who *will* offer help with wound care and even give injections. But the out-of-pocket cost for that type of service was astronomical — akin to a stay in a fancy rehabilitation facility.

I learned that most in-home nursing care involves a patient-directed companion — the equivalent of a modern lady or (man)-in-waiting. This wasn't exactly what I was looking for, but I needed help.

So, I picked a company, gave them my credit card number, and scheduled a date for their first visit for later that week.

Our House, Jim's Room

Transplant recovery is like slowly climbing a mountain back to normal. Only, when you near the summit, you realize *normal* is not as you remembered it.

Jim lost a bit of feeling in the front of his abdomen. When you touch parts of his tummy, he doesn't feel it. Obviously, the trade-off was worth it (See: living). He also had the benefit of being a lot less ticklish. But for the rest of his life, he will always need to be a bit more careful than your average person around a barbeque grill.

He also lost some feeling in the pinkie and ring fingers of his left hand. The theory was that surgical tables are narrow and Jim — at the time of his surgery — was quite wide. It was possible his left shoulder caught the lip of the table and, during his 17-hour surgery, there may have been some minor nerve damage. There was some expectation that this feeling would come back over time (spoiler alert: virtually all of it did), but for a while early in recovery it affected the strength of his grip and use of his left hand.

He also continued to have some fluid-related challenges. Jim's body was still trying to figure out its new normal. Oliver, the new liver, had recently moved in. All the other organs welcomed him in their own way. The kidneys, however, didn't trust Oliver. They were just not ready to stop working so hard. They may also have been showoffs who thought Oliver was an asshole.

While the fluid issue was no longer as dangerous as it had been before transplant surgery, it was still a challenge that required diligent management. Jim had daily weigh ins. When the liver center rang me, I'd give them all of Jim's stats, including his weight to the quarter pound. The liver center, usually via Elvia, would then give me drug-related instructions.

An oral diuretic called Lasix assisted Jim's fluid management. I reported a four-pound weight gain, I was instructed to give him more Lasix, and if I reported a six-pound loss, I would be asked to taper it off or discontinue it.

For two weeks, things went as planned. Elvia and I had our afternoon call. I dutifully reported the stats, and she gave me instructions for the drugs—a little more of this, a little less of that.

One day, I headed into Jim's room for our early morning scale time, but things did not go according to plan.

"Good morning! Let's get you out of bed."

"Something is, um, not right?" Jim said uncomfortably.

My brain immediately went to fever, rejection, etc. I pushed back the panic and shifted into my best calm voice. "Oh?"

"It's my balls."

That I had not been expecting. "What about your balls?"

"You just kind of have to check them out."

It occurred to me I was now experiencing the most unwanted conversation of every woman ever on an online dating service. I respond with: "Okay. Show me the goods."

Jim had taken to sleeping in a bathrobe. I think he found it easier than pants. Somehow, in his mind, he must have foreseen this special circumstance because:

"Oh. My. Wordy, wordy, word-word." Jim's balls were the size of a honeydew melon. This was an interesting development. "You say you woke up like this?"

"Yup. I would find this impressive if it wasn't so uncomfortable.

It was my job to report anything unusual. I thought this made the grade. I dialed Elvia on speaker.

"Elvia, I'm sorry to bother you so early, but there seems to be a bit of an issue with Jim."

"Okay. Does he have a fever?"

"No."

"Does he seem to have an infection?"

"No."

"Tell me what's going on."

"I was wondering if I could push the Lasix today?"

"How much does he weigh?"

"He hasn't been on a scale today."

"Why not?"

"Well, I haven't been able to get him on a scale."

"Why?" I sensed her losing patience with me.

"Elvia. It's his balls. They're huge."

Elvia was completely undaunted. "Is he able to stand?"

"I think so..."

"Then have him hold his balls and get on the scale. Put me on hold."

I got Jim and his balls on the scale and jotted down his new weight. He weighed exactly three pounds less than the day before.

I read today's weight to Elvia and put her on speaker.

"He weighs less than yesterday. No Lasix. We don't want to tax the kidneys."

"Is this something I should be, like, worried about?" Jim asked.

"No, it's fine. It's just the fluids in his body are shifting around."

"Will they ever, um, shift back?"

"Yes. Eventually."

"But we have an appointment later today at the liver center," I said.

I heard her sigh on the phone, and if agitation had a noise, that was it. I had disappointed Elvia. This was not good.

"Why is that a problem?"

"I have to get him into pants. What should I do?" I asked lamely.

"Make a ballamp."

"A ball lamp?"

"No, a ballamp." I heard someone calling her name in the distance. The voice sounded urgent. "I have to go. I will see you later during your visit. Tell Jim I said hello."

Jim and I looked at each other.

"I have read all the shit there is about this and I know nothing about a ball lamp. Is that a pharmacy thing?"

Jim, who was clearly far cleverer than me, asked, "Do you think she meant a ball ramp?"

"Worth a shot."

So, between morning pills and breakfast, I fashioned some washcloths and duct tape into the best damned ball ramp this town has ever seen. *Take that, Etsy!*

While there was some improvement, we still had to resort to a pair of as yet-unused-XXXXL sweatpants to accommodate Jim's cantaloupes.

We maneuvered Jim into his transport wheelchair. (Translation: He piled his balls neatly on his thighs.) To keep it classy, I added a lap blanket.

They encouraged caregivers to accompany their person into the doctor's office for the appointment, the theory being that two sets of ears were better than one and the caregiver might notice things about the patient which are of clinical interest to the doctor. I was the keeper of our questions. I added, "What about Jim's enormous balls?" to my list. I was struggling with how to frame the question in a more formal way. Maybe: "What are some practical, everyday strategies for scrotum reduction?"

But Jim, true to form, handled the situation in the most direct way possible. As we waited for a team member to call us in to the doctor's office, Jim leaned over to a fellow liver patient sitting next to him in the lobby.

I recognized the guy. He'd gotten a liver transplant about eight weeks before Jim had. As I struggled to remember his name and prepared to inquire about his health, Jim jumped in.

"So, dude. Can I ask you about your balls?"

My jaw dropped. But this guy was completely undaunted. "Yeah. Totally. What's up with your balls?"

"Man, they are huge!"

The transplant patient laughed. "Me, too. Like a pair of bocce balls for a while."

"Okay. Cool. Good to know it's not just me, you know."

Glad we got that sorted out.

CHAPTER 16: APRIL

Our House, Living Room

As Jim's health improved, so did his appetite.

The problem was this: His diet was even more restrictive than before surgery.

Jim had to continue to watch his salt. He had to obsessively watch his sugar, because glucose meters don't lie. Jim was also on the kidney diet, which meant the absence of staples like beans, potatoes, dairy, and orange juice. Oh, and grapefruit juice was now his kryptonite because it messed with drug absorption.

A bowl of minestrone, wheat toast, and a glass of Orangina was akin to a heaping bowl of rat poison.

Jim still couldn't cook for himself because of his healing chest wound. So, it was up to me to continue handling things on the culinary front.

The problem was that between administering eighteen medications at ten times throughout the day, doing blood tests, wound care, driving to and from *other* blood tests and doctor visits, speaking with pharmacists and nurses, doing mountains of laundry, ensuring the house was squeaky clean, running necessary errands, and trying my damned well best to keep up with the workload from my employer, I didn't exactly feel like putting on my jaunty little chef's hat and whipping up inspired kitchen delights.

Breakfast, lunch, and dinner kind of blended together into one big feast of culinary non-excellence. The typical meal might be a scrambled egg with applesauce and who-the-hell knew what else.

Friends thoughtfully offered to bring over food. But this would typically backfire, because people — bless their hearts — actually tried to make things taste good. One friend insisted on cooking for Jim, so I spent about fifteen minutes giving her the list of dietary restrictions. At the end, I said: "Are you sure you still want to do this?"

The next day, she showed up at our front door bearing a beautifully prepared Thanksgiving-style feast complete with roasted turkey, mashed potatoes, and a delicious marshmallow-topped sweet potato casserole.

"I didn't have time to cook, but I got this catered from a great restaurant a few towns over!" She said this to me as she waved at Jim from the front door and handed me the bag of deliciousness. I put it on the table, thanked her profusely, and then walked her out to her car. My walk back to the house was slow, as I needed to give Jim some bad news: There was not a single thing in that bag he could actually eat.

I felt like the Devil and Nurse Ratched combined. Jim deserved excellent food. But my primary job was still *"don't kill Jim."* Until he got buy in from the medical staff on a less-restrictive diet, I had to stick to the plan. Call me an overachiever, but I liked Jim not dead.

So, I stuck with the Blandy McBlanderson's medically approved diet of plain everything. Jim could manage chicken and rice a little while longer. We both could. The time for pizza was not now.

Sure, I could have whipped out the old *Yum!* book and start grating the fresh ginger. But I was tired and overwhelmed. What I wanted to do was to have someone bring me Chinese food while I stayed in bed for 24 hours straight and watched Netflix. But that wasn't an option.

When it came time for me to cook, I was well past the point of giving any fucks.

Then this happened.

I brought Jim his dinner in the living room and started to walk away to pay some medical bills.

"Hey, could you come back here a second?"

"Honey, what do you need?" I asked.

"Can I have some real dinner?"

"Excuse me?"

"Real dinner."

"What do you mean by 'real dinner?'"

"You know, like a protein and some side dishes."

I looked at his plate of broiled chicken and a melon-free, orange-free fruit cup. "Are you saying this isn't a 'real dinner?'"

"No. No, it isn't."

"It's food. That's what it is. It is food. Do you not want it?"

"I don't."

"Are you saying I could do better?"

"Yeah?"

Oh and didn't that hit a nerve.

"I'm leaving." I announced.

"Where are you going?"

"Out."

"Out where?"

"I don't know. I guess to get you some real Goddamned dinner!" I grabbed a coat, phone and keys and stomped out the front door, slamming it behind me for good measure.

I thought a moment and poked my head back in.

"I will have my phone and will not be far away. I need a half hour. Call if there's a genuine emergency, okay?"

I re-slammed the door.

I re-opened the door.

"Oh. And go fuck yourself."

I slammed the door again.

No one can inspire such spirited loathing like one's spouse.

It had been 10 straight months of awful. Would things ever get better? Could we ever just be normal people doing normal things again?

I wanted to get in the car and just drive and not stop. I just wanted to get away—far, far away—from Jim. From this. But being both exhausted and unimaginative, I got as far as the Senior Center parking lot less than a mile away and parked my car.

I had hoped to spend 20 minutes reading a book and then calm down enough to reclaim my patience and go home. But when I reached into my purse for my book, there was only the big bag of prescriptions I'd picked up the day before. My book was on the dining room table, right where I had left it before my trip to the pharmacy, to make room for the pills.

And then the emotional dam broke.

An angry cry is not like a regular cry. With an angry cry, the tears feel as if they're punching through your tear ducts to flow down your face. I started making noises — those keening sounds you usually only hear from scenery-chewing actors.

I was sitting behind the wheel of my parked car, crying and rocking. I then looked up and saw that the view from my car was of the adjacent elementary school parking lot. I saw a kid on the swing being pushed by her mom. Crying then became outright weeping because I was further reminded of all the things we didn't have.

When your loved one receives the gift of life, this act hammers gratitude in to you. You should be grateful for the gift. (He was. We were.) You should be thankful your life was spared. (He was. We were.) You should feel blessed you are able to go on. (He does. We do.)

But it's complicated.

He survived. But maybe *we* didn't.

In sickness and in health meant you should stay together during the bad times, but it said nothing about actually liking each other.

Jim was no longer my husband. He was my patient.

I realized a bunch of little things had been piling up: Jim had stopped asking how I was feeling. He didn't ask what I wanted to watch on TV. Our relationship had become transactional. Get this. Do that.

We loved each other. We just didn't like each other much anymore. There were no guidebooks for this. I was at a loss. But, I needed to address the more immediate problem: Jim needed to eat and was clearly unsatisfied with the menu—and I was unsatisfied with him being unsatisfied with the menu.

Cooking classes were out. Dinner at a restaurant was out. Even takeout was out.

Then, I had an idea. I wiped my wet face with the back of my coat sleeve, started up the engine and turned the car towards home.

I parked in the driveway and walked through the front door and right up to the recliner.

"I'm going to get your shoes and a coat. We're going out."

"Where?"

"It's a surprise."

"Are you taking me out back to shoot me?"

"What? No. It's not far. But, finish this fruit cup first. You will need to take pills in the next hour."

He chugged it.

"There was a spoon."

"This sounds like an adventure. Why wait?" I helped put on his shoes, grabbed his elbows and hoisted him out of the chair. For the first time in a long time, Jim looked really excited.

In 15 minutes, we arrive at the destination—the big box food store down Route 1.

I handed him a disposable medical mask to put on.

"Let's do some shopping. Together."

"Really?"

"Yup."

He smiled, "Like, a date?"

"Yup. Like a real date."

I had been sticking to grocery stores close to home for the past few months, so I hadn't been here in a while. I vaguely remembered them having motorized carts.

"So, I'm going to drop you out front, okay? Then I will park the car and help you inside."

It took me a while to find a spot—way in the back of the lot. By the time I walked up to the store and inside, Jim had not only found the carts but was receiving enthusiastic instructions on how to use one from one of the greeters at the door. I had joined them at the end of the lesson.

"So, you just unplug and go."

"Where do we pay the rental fee?"

"What do you mean?"

"Yes, how much for the cart?"

"To buy it? You'd really need to talk to Customer Service about that."

"No, I mean to drive around the store and get stuff."

"Oh! There's no charge for that."

I felt as if I was in a different dimension. Meanwhile, Jim had looked at me like I was nuts. Was he in on this *free-carts* thing this entire time?

Jim drove with the proficiency of a Formula One driver, deftly maneuvering around pallets of animal crackers and early Easter candy displays. It only then occurred to me he hadn't been behind a wheel in a while.

His mask also gave him a bit of a bank robber quality.

"Now just try to keep up with meeeeee!" He sped down the long aisle at a brisk three miles-per-hour.

I yelled after him. "Go find us some real dinner!"

That he did. He found so many dinners and lunches and snacks that his basket overflowed, and I had to go back to the front of the store for a full-sized cart.

Jim approached his dietary restrictions with a good bit of creativity. He'd found some breaded fish fillets comfortably within his salt range and then some fruit salsa to go with them. He also found some exotic rice varieties which could go right into the microwave.

Sure, he still had to avoid things like canned soup and potato chips, but Jim opened my eyes to a complete world of things I didn't even know he liked.

He cruised and shopped while I browsed in a separate part of the store. It occurred to me this was the first recreational shopping I had done in a while. I actually spent a full ten minutes choosing between two different types of deodorant.

As I wandered back with the lavender-scented loot in my hand, I spied Jim at the flower case. He was talking to one of the store employees. She handed him a bouquet from the top row, which he carefully deposited in his cart.

I saw him head for the checkout. I pulled my cart up behind him.

"Those are some lovely flowers you got there."

"They're for the cats. You know, for our reunion," he smiled. Doctors just gave us the okay to spring them from their basement bachelor pad.

"They're really pretty, but we're not supposed to have flowers in the house because, you know, immunities."

"They're for your office. I don't go in there, right?"

"No, but..."

"Why are you killing the romance here?"

Exactly one hour later, I heard the timer on the fish fillets go off as I was arranging the flowers in a vase in the office. As I walked into the kitchen to get dinner ready, Jim was finding a movie for us both to watch.

We were about to enjoy our first real dinner *and* a movie for the first time in a long time.

In the Air, Far Away from New Jersey

The day of reckoning had arrived.

I was leaving for a week-long business trip, and I was a wreck.

I wasn't even sure what I packed in my suitcase. There may have been twelve pairs of pants and no underwear. I had no idea.

I'd hit a last-minute snag the prior week when my mother had a health complication of her own. Her stomach ailment from a few weeks earlier had worsened. She spent some time in the hospital and was now recuperating at home. My mom felt wretched. She needed rest and healing. There was also enough of a possibility of Jim catching what she had that it was a dangerous move to put both of them in a room together. So now, Mom and Dad were out of the caregiver mix.

The revised plan would involve a rotating team of friends and visiting nurses. During my time away, Jim's care schedule looked like this:

Jim's friend Jay would fly down from Canada and spend the first few days of my trip at our house. His visit and my departure would overlap. That way, I could talk him through Jim's schedule, pills, meal plan, important contact information, and what to do in case of emergency.

After Jay departed, a mix of visiting nurses and some local friends who'd offered to do shifts would cover us for the remaining three days. Jim would also have his cell phone with him at all times. If he could not reach a friend, the backup plan would be for Jim to call the local rescue squad for help. He also had every number of any doctor he'd ever visited programmed into his phone.

Before my departure, I stocked the refrigerator and pantry full of Jim-friendly foods. I organized a week's worth of pills, as well as a backup week of pills, just in case. I cleaned everything within an inch of its life and made sure there was a month's worth of clean clothes, linens, and towels in reserve. Jim and his wellness crew were to send me frequent health updates via text.

With the flurry of preparations, I barely remembered I was going on a trip until the plane was in the sky.

When I got off the plane, I immediately checked for text updates. There were none.

Me: Jim, you okay?
Jim: All good. Jay and I are watching Netflix.
Me: Are you taking your pills?
Jim: Yes.
Me: Is Jay feeding you?
Jim: I fed myself, actually. Grownup, remember?
Me: Love you.
Jim: Love you, too. I'm fine. Now go run a company.

I kept checking my texts throughout the day and into the next morning. Still nothing.

Me: All good?
Jim: All good!
Me: Okay. TTYL. Mind texting me an update later?
Jim: Sure.

Later there was no update except a picture of Jim with the cats entitled, *"Freeeeeeeeddddddooooommmmm!!!"*

After again being allowed upstairs, they ambushed Jim. He lavished them with attention.

Me: Remember to use sanitizer!
Jim: I would, but Cato can't open it for me. No thumbs.
Me: I am serious. Wash your damned hands.

No texts meant I could give my full attention to work, and it felt fantastic. I was putting my time and energy into activities that had absolutely nothing to do with my relationship. My brain felt as if someone had opened the windows and let in the fresh air and sunshine.

It did, however, take some discipline not to check my phone incessantly. I managed to avoid looking at my texts for a full four hours. When I looked again—nothing.

Me: Checking in.
Jim: All good here. Love you.

And that's how it went. For days. Cat pictures and *"all goods."* I even tried a workaround by reaching out to friends.

Me: Hiya! You stopped by to see Jim yet?
Lisa: Yeah. I went by this morning.
Me: How was he?
Lisa: All good!
Me: Thanks for stopping by. I appreciate it.
Lisa: No worries. He can also call me anytime he needs something.
Me: Seriously. You are awesome. Are you really sure he's okay?
Lisa: LOL. He's all good. I promise.

And then:

Me: Thanks for stopping by and seeing Jim.
Reagan: Yeah, I went by tonight. He looked good!
Me: Would you say he looked, "All good?"
Reagan: Yup. All good.
Me: Seriously?!?
Reagan: I'm serious. He is all good.

Never play a player. If Reagan was going vague, something was up.

I called Jim.

"Hey, what's up?"

"What's up with you?"

"All good here. How goes it with you?"

"I would say I'm 'all good' except..."

"That's the door. Hold on a second." I heard him yell, "Hey, could you just leave it? Thanks! I take a while to get to the door. I left a gratuity on the card, man!"

"And who was that?"

"The pizza guy."

"What?!?"

"Dominoes posts a really detailed menu online, right? If I ask for barbeque sauce and half cheese, I can keep it below my salt count. I've never been much of a fan before, but I have a newfound fondness for the stuff."

"Oh...that's good. That's really good."

"I gotta go. It can take me a while to get to the door, and I want to eat it while it's hot, you know. Hey, I can't wait to see you tomorrow."

"Same here. Love you."

The next day I opened the front door and dragged my luggage into the living room to find Jim there alone watching TV.

"Come on over and give me a hug!" He said.

I looked around. "So, where's the nurse?"

"Oh, I sent her home."

"I really shouldn't bring all these germs into the house. Let me spray my bag with some Lysol and then throw myself into the shower."

"I have a better idea. How about you skip the Lysol, hop in the shower, and then go grab a glass of wine. I'd love to hear how your week went."

"Oh, okay. Do you need anything?"

"Not now. I am all good."

I returned fifteen minutes later, wearing a robe, with my hair wrapped in a towel, and a healthy-sized glass of Pinot Grigio in my hand. When I plopped down on the couch, Jim asked about my week. I walked through the usual work dramas — the ups and the downs. He listened thoughtfully and asked questions for the next hour. When I was all talked out about work stuff, I shifted my attention back to him.

"So, about your week..."

"I survived."

"Clearly." I raised my eyebrows critically.

"Well, it was not without its complications." There it was. Jim then finally opened up about the meandering, epic, weird story of the past few days.

When Jay had visited, they'd watched a ton of sci-fi movies. During this time, Jim, with Jay's full endorsement, rediscovered takeout.

Post Jay's departure, Jim had cancelled visiting nurse services. He got tired of having a new person at the house every day that we would need to manage. He also missed his privacy.

Then there was Reagan. Unable to get a sitter for Daniel, her foster son, she'd brought him along with her to the house. Upon arrival, he'd touched every item in the house. After doing so, he loudly announced, "I gotta take a shit," and started heading toward Jim's bathroom. When Reagan saw the look of horror in Jim's eyes, she blocked Daniel's path, shooed him out to the car, and floored it to her house across down.

Then, there was Lisa, who had a tough time getting to the house that week. Stuff had happened with her kids and the week had gotten away from her. Hearing her struggle to make it all work, Jim had insisted he was fine and sent her on her way.

"I just had a good handle on things, you know. Why burden anyone if I had it covered?" He paused. "I can do this, you know."

"What?"

"Living."

"I know." I said, not really sure I believed it.

"You can let go now. Not all the way. Just a little. Because you have to do this living thing, too, you know."

"I know."

I reached for his hand.

"Did you sanitize that?" Jim asked mischievously.

I rolled my eyes. "You know, we make a pretty good team."

"That we do."

"We need a team name. You know, like a band name."

"Can it have robots in it?"

"How about "Some Assembly Required?""

"Sounds about right."

"I couldn't agree more."

EPILOGUE

We decided not to do gifts this year. Nothing ever really tops living.

Instead, we spent a day out together and took the train into the city. Christmas was still six days away, but the city had already been celebrating for weeks now. We were celebrating, too.

We stopped for coffee and then walked over to see the tree. Even on a workday morning, the place was packed. Clearly, we were not the only ones with this bright idea. Perhaps the weather had something to do with it. Jacket and hat weather, crisp and cold, but with the sun bright.

We openly wondered why we didn't come to the city more often. Being from New Jersey, we were close enough to make the trip, but far enough away to make it seem foreign and a little magical.

I kept checking my watch, and every time I did, Jim looked at me and smiled.

"I think I'm just so worried about being late."

"I'm fine with being early."

"Me too."

Jim took my hand and we walked up the crowded street, making a left on 51st.

On a gold awning, in white letters, we saw just what we'd been looking for:

Le Bernardin.

After nearly five years, it was time.

"You ready?" I asked.

"Yeah, I am."

AFTERWORD

As I clean up this manuscript for final submission to my publisher, I write to you from bed.

A month ago my gynecologist called to tell me I have thyroid cancer. (You may wonder about the gynecologist part of that last sentence, but I best save the explanation, in case I write another book.) A week ago I had surgery to remove the offending gland and a few lymph nodes for good measure. Today I bear a fresh surgical scar on my neck, the likes of which Sweeney Todd would find impressive.

Experiencing illness from the patient side of things brings new perspective. I now know the creeping numbness you feel when you have a sickness time or prescription medicine alone won't fix. I've felt the acute fear of knowing I could not handle this alone. Most important of all, I experienced the immeasurable comfort of knowing I wouldn't have to.

Jim's first words upon hearing my diagnosis were: "We got this."

Yeah, we do.

POSTSCRIPT

Since the time of Jim's transplant, the Model for End-stage Liver Disease score has been updated to include consideration of sodium levels. In January 2016, Model for End-stage Liver Disease and Sodium (MELD-Na) was introduced as the new standard for liver allocation. Studies have shown that it has significantly decreased waitlist mortality.

For the latest information on advancements in organ allocation and transplantation in the United States, visit the United Network for Organ Sharing (UNOS) web site http://unos.org.

REGISTER TO GIVE THE GIFT OF LIFE
Make your next minute matter.

Register as an organ and tissue donor and help save a life!
Registration takes less than one minute with 3 easy ways to sign up:
Phone Health App: iPhone users can quickly and easily join the National Donate Life Registry using the Health app
Online at RegisterMe.org (mobile-friendly)
Visit your local Motor Vehicle Agency
By registering your decision to be an organ, eye and tissue donor in the National Donate Life Registry, you are helping to save lives and give hope to the 110,000 people in the United States currently waiting for lifesaving organ transplants. Thousands more people are in need of tissue or corneal transplants to restore health. One donor can save and heal more than 75 lives.

ACKNOWLEDGEMENTS

To the donor who gave Jim the gift of life: While your life was too short, your kindness is eternal.

To every doctor, surgeon, nurse and staff member of the University Hospital Center for Advanced Liver Diseases and Transplantation: You are in the business of making miracles happen. Thank you for being so committed to Jims care and treating us like family.

To NJ Sharing Network, Donate Life America, and the United Network for Organ Sharing (UNOS): Thank you for spreading the life-saving message of organ donation and for making the gift of life possible.

To Dr. Thomas Starzl: Thank you for demonstrating to the world that liver transplants are possible and extending the lives of countless people because of it.

To Mom and Dad: Thank you for raising a resilient kid and being there for Jim all the times I couldn't. I love you to bits.

To friends Rachel, Josh, Mike, and Laurie: You helped during the times most absent of hope. Thanks for helping to carry Jim and us across the finish line.

To my entire work family, and most especially Bel, Claudio, Phil, Mel, Molly, Rick, Becky, and Henry: I will never forget your support during an incomparably difficult time. Thank you.

To Mary Ellen, Alessandro, and Marnee: Thank you for the needed nudge that made me to write this book.

To Cathie, Lisa, and all my sisters: Your encouragement means the world. I am so very grateful for you.

To patients currently on the organ transplant waiting list: Your bravery inspires us all. May you get the call soon.

ABOUT THE AUTHOR

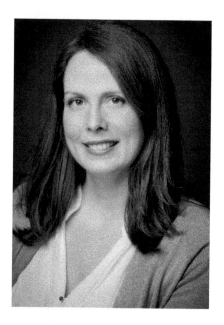

TJ Condon is a marketing executive and published writer. She is a passionate advocate for organ donation, is an active volunteer with NJ Sharing Network (Donate Life America affiliate) and has served as a board member for a number of non-profit organizations. TJ holds a Master of Communication and Information Studies degree from Rutgers University and a Bachelor of Arts degree in English from Dickinson College.

NOTE FROM THE AUTHOR

Word-of-mouth is crucial for any author to succeed. If you enjoyed *Some Assembly Required*, please leave a review online — anywhere you are able. Even if it's just a sentence or two. It would make all the difference and would be very much appreciated.

Thanks!
TJ Condon

Thank you so much for reading one
of our **Medical Non-Fiction** novels.
If you enjoyed the experience, please check out our recommended
title for your next great read!

A Red Door by Kathryn Jarvis

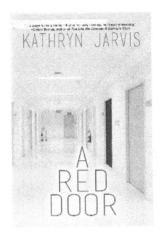

"...a page-turning memoir that is not only riveting,
but heart-wrenching."
–Embry Burrus, author of
The Life We Choose: A Sibling's Story

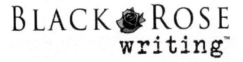

CPSIA information can be obtained
at www.ICGtesting.com
Printed in the USA
FSHW020505240521
81636FS

9 781684 337361